Slimming by Numbers

Numerical tools to get you the body you want

Dr Jeff Pursglov

Dedication

To all of you who refuse to lie down

Contents

Chapter 1: The body you want

"Do the thing and you will have the power" (Ralph Waldo Emerson)

How you will benefit from this book

It is so easy to lose weight and change your shape! All you need to do is to watch your diet and get plenty of exercise. What could be simpler? Well, you and I both know that it is not that straightforward, and anyone who tells you that it is just does not understand the complexity of the situation that you are in. Your complicated problem needs powerful tools to fix it.

Your situation is like that of a business that is in poor shape. The CEO of a struggling company knows that improving its performance is simply a matter of reducing costs and increasing income: but the difficulty lies in knowing how to achieve this. Fortunately, several robust tools and techniques have been developed over the years, by some of the best brains around, to enable businesses to work out the underlying reasons for their poor performance and to take steps to improve it.

You too can now benefit from these tools, because in this book I will show you how to use the best of these tried and tested business techniques, firstly to:

- Identify what it is that you are doing now, or have done in the past, that has caused your current shape

And then, secondly to:

- Do things differently to get a vastly improved shape

These tools work for businesses that want to get into shape, and they will work for you, even if all your previous attempts have failed.

Possibly you are very overweight: you seem to have tried everything, but you just cannot change things. Or maybe you are already in reasonable shape, but want to look above average. Or perhaps your current shape lies somewhere in between these two extremes. No matter what shape you are in now, you can use the tools in this book to make things better.

In the following pages I am going to show you how to get the body you want by using the tools and techniques of business performance management. I have done it (and there is nothing special about me), and so you can do it. Although it has taken me a long time to get this together and to put it down on paper, all it will take you is the time you spend in reading and acting on the contents of this book.

The birth of this book

The seeds of this book were sown when I was fired from my job on an icy day in February, 1995. I was aged 38 and living in Cumbria: a remote part of the UK, with few employment opportunities. Up to then, I had tried to keep reasonably fit and healthy, but I smoked a pipe and probably drank too much. To be honest, I wasn't in very good shape.

At the time of losing my job I felt that it was a disastrous event, but I now realize that it was an opportunity to assess my lifestyle, improve it, and achieve new things. I had two options. The first one was to wallow in self-pity, become bitter to those around me, blame everyone but myself for my predicament, and to give up on life. The second option was to develop a positive attitude, accept total responsibility for my situation, decide what I really wanted out of life, and to make good use of the mass of spare time that I now had available to achieve it. I chose the second option. As a result, within four years, I was able to transform my body (without the use of performance-enhancing drugs) to win the senior-level Mr. York bodybuilding competition, and be awarded an MBA by a prestigious university. During the following seven years I became an expert in the tools of business performance management by publishing papers, delivering speeches at international conferences, and applying my skills in new jobs. I also won many more bodybuilding competitions, culminating in the Mr. Britain seniors' title in 2006. These events were not disconnected, because I used what I had learned and discovered about business performance management to change the shape of my body. I wanted a hard, rugged, muscular physique and I used these tools to get one.

I also benefited enormously from talking to other top athletes: in the gym, at competitions and via on line discussion forums. I discovered what made these people tick: how they trained, what they ate and how they motivated themselves.

When I changed my shape and became well known, I found more and more people asking for my advice on how to improve their own shape. Sometimes I would be approached in the gym, sometimes at work, sometimes by e-mail and sometimes even in the aisles of the local supermarket! If I was asked just to put together a diet and/or a workout routine, I would usually direct the enquirer to some of the excellent books or websites that cover just those topics. I did not believe that I could add much value to what was already available to them by scribbling something down on a sheet of paper. On the other hand, if someone asked me more generally to help them to get into shape, then I would spend more time with them. These individuals understood that getting into shape involved more than someone simply telling them what to eat and how to exercise, because if it was that easy, then they would already have done it.

At first, my advice would be sound, but somewhat haphazard, in that I would use a mixture of the business techniques that I had used to change my own shape. However, since setting up my own personal training business, I have developed a much more structured approach to the adaptation and application of these techniques. Indeed, the course that led to my qualification in personal training reinforced my conviction that there was a desperate need for techniques and frameworks with which to analyze and improve clients' lifestyles, in order to enable them to get the body they desired. Before this book, my only means of enabling individuals to use these tools to change their shape was by sitting alongside and talking things through with them. With this book I can now help so many others, especially you!

How this book differs from all others

I am sure you already know that the two main things that count towards getting into shape are:

- Food intake
- Exercise

However, I have not written this book to tell you what to eat or how to exercise, (and not just because the chances are that you already know these things anyway!). What I am going to do is to equip you with the necessary tools, and the knowledge of how to use them, so that you can alter whatever it is that has caused your shape. You will end up with a solution to your problems that is tailor-made to your situation, not something that is supposed to work for everyone. This is crucial, because each and every one of you reading this book will be relatively rich or poor in different things, such as:

- Favourable genetics
- Motivation to change your shape
- Time available to exercise, or to prepare meals
- Availability of fitness equipment, gym membership or even a personal trainer
- Knowledge of how your body responds to diet and exercise
- Support of family and friends
- Energy to exercise
- Self-confidence to do new and different things

So, this book is not about new exercises or novel diets. Many excellent books have already been written on those topics and I expect that you, like me, will have read a lot of them. Visit any news stand and you will see rows of magazines covering the whole spectrum of subjects, from the latest 'miracle' diets used by celebrities to drop a dress size or two, to the sure-fire way for a man to get that all important six-pack in a matter of weeks. There is also a massive amount of free, first-class information on the Internet. So, despite all this, why are so many people out of shape?

Why you are the shape you are

Assuming that you do not suffer from a debilitating illness or injury then, for your age, you are the shape you are today due to the combined effects of the genetic make-up of your body (i.e., your genotype), and what you have done to your body in the past. Clearly, you cannot alter either the traits that you inherited from your parents or your age, so the only way that you can change your shape is to treat your body differently compared to how you have done in the past.

If you are unhappy with your current shape, then you must take some responsibility for that. Do not feel guilty: just accept responsibility. You must not blame circumstances, bad luck, your partner, your work, your family etc. Accepting this is a revelation, because with responsibility comes power. Once you accept that it is your own actions that have contributed to your current shape, it follows that you also accept that you can change your shape, to make it what you want it to be. That is all there is to it.

Now, I know that if you are seriously out of shape, then you may not agree with the preceding paragraph. You may believe that your shape is primarily determined by your genetics and that, if you have a so called 'obesity gene' in your make up, then you are doomed to live in a pear-shaped body until the day you die. Well, all that I can do is to re-iterate that, although your genotype may have given you the propensity to be overweight, the shape of your body is influenced massively by how you treat it. Although you may have a genetic predisposition towards a certain body shape, the fact that each succeeding generation is heavier than the last proves that changes in our bodies' environment are playing the key role.

My genotype certainly affected how I had to train to become a champion bodybuilder. My legs are naturally long and skinny, and so I had to really bomb them in the gym for them to grow to match my upper body. On the other hand, I had no problems in building a great back and terrific abs.

So, at the end of the day, although your genotype is going to make it relatively easier or harder for you to change your shape, it is not going to make it impossible for you to do so. Also, you should remember that, if you were once 'in shape', your genetics will not prevent you from re-gaining that shape.

Activities above all

Just in case you are still in any doubt, I want to emphasize that the only way you can change your shape is by living your life differently from how you live it now. Do not be overwhelmed by that statement of fact: the tools in this book will show you the changes that you must make. However, it does not matter how many times you work through this book, unless you act on what these tools are telling you, then your shape will not improve: achievement comes from the doing, not from the reading. You will need to stop some current activities, and start some new activities; otherwise, your shape will probably not just stay as it is: it will move even further away from the body you want.

The tools featured

We start in **Chapter 2** with the technique of Force Field analysis from the USA. This tool identifies the positive and negative forces that are driving your current shape to get better or worse. It deals mainly with actions and circumstances, and it is a good, simple tool to start with, especially as the case study that we use does not involve working out in the gym!

The next three chapters feature quality improvement tools that the Japanese used to revolutionize their manufacturing industries after World War 2. These techniques (Relationship, Ishikawa, and Tree diagrams) enabled the Japanese to become the dominant force worldwide in sectors such as automobiles and electrical goods. Each of them uses a different approach, enabling us to delve deeper and identify the underlying reasons (such as your knowledge, attitude, and habits) for your current shape. In **Chapter 5** you will see that I have turned the Tree diagram on its head, so that we can use it more as a tool to propel you towards your ideal shape.

Chapter 6 introduces the technique of Benchmarking, developed originally by the Xerox Corporation in the USA. This is the first technique that requires you to collect data and compare yourself with others. However, the emphasis here is not about measuring your shape and comparing it with others, so much as identifying and recording best practice in the processes that determine body shapes.

Chapters 7 and **8** are devoted to Results Based Accountability and the Balanced Scorecard. These are more recent techniques originating from the USA. Both are excellent tools for developing plans to enable you to get the shape you want. They are both quantitative, requiring the identification and measurement of key Performance Indicators (PIs).

So, in terms of complexity, I rate these tools as follows:

- **Foundation level**: Force Field analysis and Relationship diagrams
- **Intermediate level**: Ishikawa diagrams, Tree diagrams and Benchmarking
- **Advanced level**: Results Based Accountability and Balanced Scorecard

Figure 1.1 shows, for each tool, whether or not you will need to take measurements, and/or involve others.

<u>Figure 1.1</u>

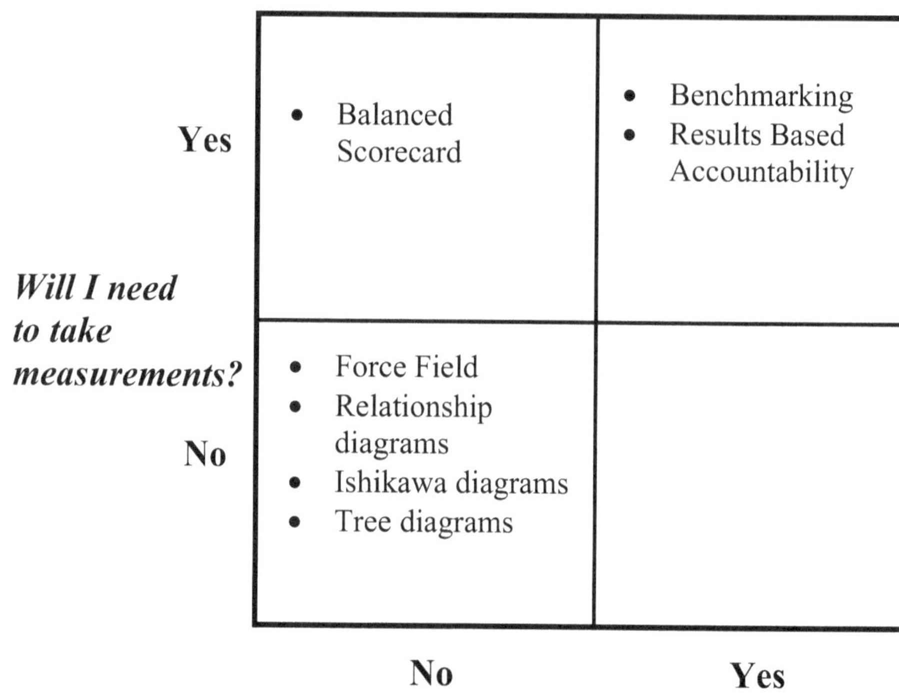

The case studies

I have illustrated each of the tools with a case study. Although the individuals in the case studies are fictitious, they have all been developed from clients of mine that have used these techniques successfully. You will read the stories of:

- Bob, a 45-year-old executive who had gained a lot of weight since his divorce (Force Field analysis)
- Naomi, a 35-year-old stay-at-home mother of three, who went up three dress sizes after the birth of her children (Relationship diagrams)

- Emily, a 32-year-old solicitor whose hectic lifestyle prevented her eating and exercising properly (Ishikawa diagrams)
- Amber, 26 years old and plump since puberty, who felt that she was missing out dating attractive men because of her shape (Tree diagrams)
- Graham, strong but stocky at 33 years of age, whose weight was starting to have a bad effect on his health (Benchmarking)
- Clive, a 55-year-old owner of his own company, who needed to lose around 20 lbs to enjoy his imminent retirement (Results Based Accountability)
- Wendy, a 45-year-old nurse, who had started binge eating and drinking following the death of her husband, but was now determined to get back into shape for her daughter's wedding (Balanced Scorecard)

How to use this book

This is a practical book. Its focus is on working with these tools and applying them both to yourself, and to your own individual circumstances. You do not have to know a thing about business to use these tools. Although I describe briefly the business background of each tool at the beginning of each chapter, you can skip this if you want. All you need to work through these techniques is:

- A pencil and sharpener
- An eraser
- A ruler
- Some sticky notes or 5" x 3" cards
- Plenty of plain A4 and a few sheets of graph paper

Most of these techniques were developed before the advent of desktops, laptops, and tablets, and so none of them require that you must use a computer. However, for some of them, the use of a computer will make things tidier. Or maybe you would just prefer to use a computer regardless. If so, that is fine. My own preference is to begin using the tools with pencil and paper (because this helps me to be more creative) and then to put my work onto a computer once I have finished thinking things through.

Although all these tools are fun to use, you will probably find that you particularly like one or two of them. As I showed in **Figure 1.1**, Benchmarking and Results Based Accountability do need input from others. You can choose to use the rest of the tools either by yourself, or with friends who also want to improve their shape. Working in a group can often give you fresh insights and more ideas, but remember that the outcome for each member of the group will be different, unless you are identical twins and have led exactly the same lifestyle so far! Also, you must be completely truthful when using these techniques. If you drink a couple of glasses of wine, or eat a lot of chocolates most nights, then you owe it to yourself to say so. It is no good whatsoever kidding yourself otherwise. So, do not work in a group if you think that feeling self-conscious or embarrassed is going to prevent you from telling the truth, because in that situation you will not reap the benefits that you deserve from these techniques.

In terms of identifying why you are the shape you are, and what you need to do to change it, then each of these tools should come up with broadly similar answers. If you find that you are getting markedly different answers from some of the tools, then you are probably doing something wrong, such as not being completely honest with yourself. However, you should not expect to get identical answers from each technique. This is because the management theory behind each of them is different, their original intended purpose is different, and using them is more of an art than a precise science.

Chapter 2: May the force be with you
(Force Field analysis)

"If you want to truly understand something, try to change it"
(Kurt Lewin)

Business background

The psychologist Kurt Lewin (1890-1947) was born in Germany, but he came to the United States in 1932, ending his career as the director of the Research Center for Group Dynamics at the Massachusetts Institute of Technology. Lewin hypothesised that any given situation in an organization is the result of two opposing sets of forces: the *driving forces* (trying to bring about change) and the *restraining forces* (trying to prevent change). For an organization to change, managers must identify these forces, and then reduce the restraining forces whilst increasing the strength of the driving forces.

For example, the manager of a bakery used Force Field analysis to find that the expected increase in profits resulting from:

- Cheaper imported ingredients due to a favourable exchange rate
- Greater production following investment in new machinery

Was being hindered by

- High distribution costs caused by small orders
- Low selling prices because of a bland product range

Key features

Strengths

- Foundation level: the simplest of all the tools

- No measuring or data are required
- It is very visual
- There is no need to involve others
- This tool shows clearly the dynamic nature of the factors that determine your shape
- It quickly leads to an action plan with which to change your shape

But bear in mind

- This tool is not good at identifying the underlying psychological causes of your current shape
- It is not a tool designed to monitor your progress towards your new shape

The technique explained

Draw a straight line (called the *continuum*) that represents all of the possible shapes of your body, ranging from your worst possible shape to your best possible or ideal shape. Place a mark where you feel that your current shape lies on the continuum (**Figure 2.1**).

Next, think about how your shape has changed over the last year or so. This is your shape's *direction of travel*. Has your shape stayed the same (**Figure 2.2**), is it deteriorating (**Figure 2.3**), or is it improving (**Figure 2.4**)? To help you to decide upon this, you can just consider simple things, such as your clothes size. If you have other information available, such as records of your weight or percentage body fat, you can look at that too. However, perhaps the most important factor is going to be how you feel about the shape of your body. Have you been stuck for some time now with a shape that you dislike? Do you feel that you have made improvements to your shape, or is it going from bad to worse? Once you have decided on the direction of travel, show it on the continuum.

<u>Figure 2.1</u>

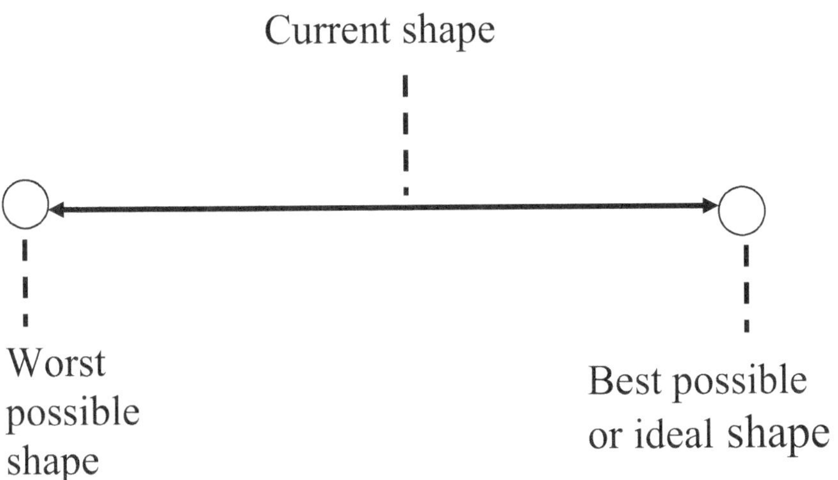

<u>Figure 2.2</u>

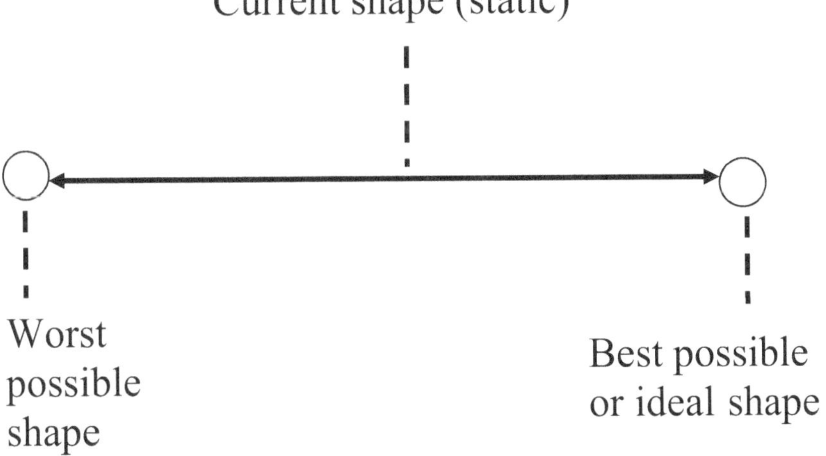

<u>Figure 2.3</u>

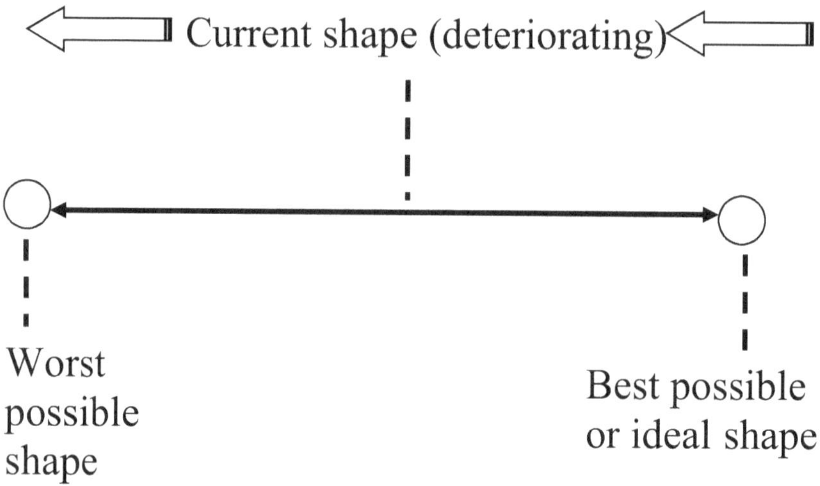

<u>Figure 2.4</u>

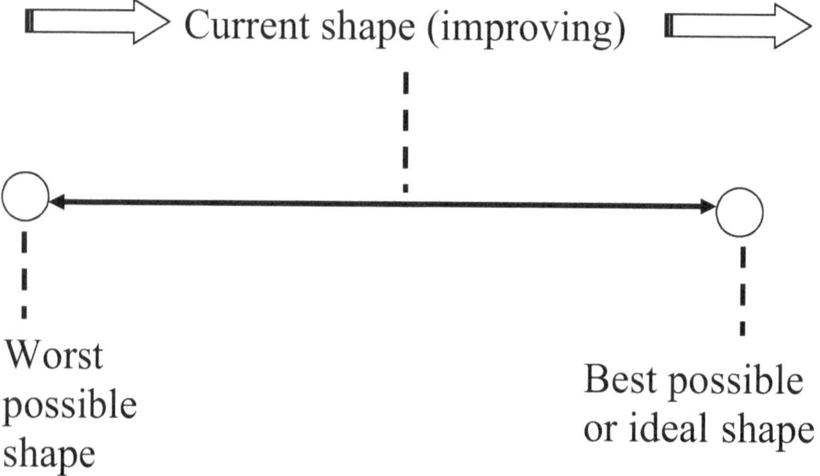

I now want you to visualize the shape of your body as being the result of many different forces acting upon it, pushing and pulling it in or out of shape. If you decided earlier that your current shape is static, then the forces pushing to improve your shape are balanced equally by other forces pushing it to get worse. In this situation, we can say that the two sets of opposing forces are in *equilibrium*. If your shape is deteriorating, this means that the forces pushing it to worsen are overpowering the forces working to improve your shape. If your shape is improving, the reverse is true. So, what you must do is to identify, and then estimate, the strength of the forces driving your body shape from both directions along the continuum. You can then develop a plan to increase the total strength of the forces pushing to improve your shape, and to weaken the forces resisting them.

As with all of the tools in this book, I will explain how to use it by working through a real-life example.

Bob's story

Bob, aged 45, manages a car leasing business. He and his wife divorced two years ago, and he now lives on his own. His ex-wife will tell you that she divorced him because he thought more about his job than he did about her. Bob has gained weight since his divorce. He now weighs 210 pounds compared to only 180 pounds a few years ago, and he is still getting heavier.

Bob rarely eats breakfast, preferring to get up and drive straight to the office. On arrival, he drinks the first of his six daily cups of coffee. By mid-morning, he needs a couple of chocolate biscuits to keep him going. Most days, he has a calorie-rich, three-course business lunch with suppliers or customers. On the way home from work, Bob often picks up a takeaway and washes it down with a few bottles of beer whilst watching television. Bob does not have the energy to do much else, and so he employs a gardener for a couple of hours each week to mow the lawns and tidy the garden.

Bob's exercise is confined to weekends. He plays a round of golf with his friends and business associates on both Saturdays and Sundays and, if he is not driving, he usually enjoys a few drinks at the 'nineteenth hole'.

His motivation for wanting to escape his shape is that he is becoming increasingly self-conscious about the image that he projects to customers and colleagues. Bob thinks that he will be passed over for promotion if he does not do something about his shape.

Before he turned 40, Bob used to work out a couple of times a week. So, three months ago, he tried going to his local gym at weekends. This soon stopped because he did not enjoy it, especially as it clashed with his golf.

Bob's Force Field

After thinking about his lifestyle, Bob identified just one positive force compared to eight negative ones acting on his shape. He drew them as arrows on his Force Field diagram (**Figure 2.5**). Next, Bob estimated how powerful each of these forces was, by scoring them from **1** (weak) to **5** (strong). The resulting Force Field was **4:26** against his shape: little wonder that his shape had deteriorated so much and so rapidly!

We can calculate the relative strength of the negative forces using this formula:

$$\% \text{ superiority of negative forces} = ((\text{-ve forces} - \text{+ve forces}) \div \text{+ve forces}) \times 100$$

So,

$$\% \text{ superiority of negative forces} = ((26 - 4) \div 4) \times 100$$

$$= 550\%$$

Figure 2.5

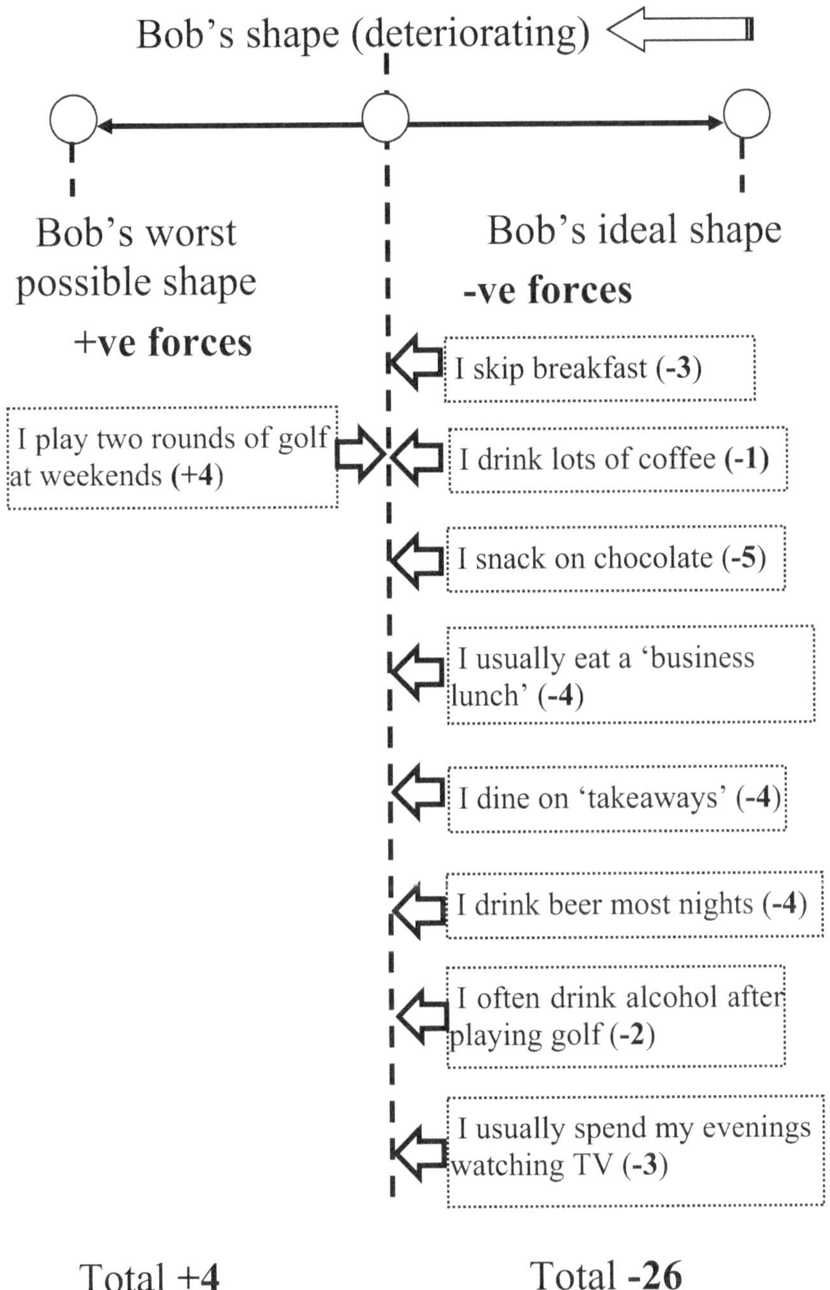

Bob's shape (deteriorating)
Bob's worst possible shape
+ve forces
Bob's ideal shape
-ve forces
I skip breakfast (-3)
I play two rounds of golf at weekends (+4)
I drink lots of coffee (-1)
I snack on chocolate (-5)
I usually eat a 'business lunch' (-4)
I dine on 'takeaways' (-4)
I drink beer most nights (-4)
I often drink alcohol after playing golf (-2)
I usually spend my evenings watching TV (-3)
Total +4
Total -26

For Bob to halt the continuing worsening of his shape, and then allow it to start to improve, he had to figure out how to get the total scores of the positive forces to outweigh the total scores of the negative forces. Bob's situation was dire, but not hopeless. After a couple of 'brainstorming' sessions, and scribbling of possible solutions, Bob decided on an action plan that he felt was sufficiently realistic for him to implement and live with. Bob decided to do the following:

- Set his alarm for 15 minutes earlier in the morning to give him time to eat a bowl of muesli for breakfast (benefit **minus 3** from negative forces)
- Drink four large glasses of water a day from the cooler outside his office: however, he will then still allow himself to drink as much coffee as he wanted (benefit: **plus 2** on positive forces)
- Put a fruit bowl on his desk and load it with bananas, oranges, and apples to snack on in place of chocolate bars (benefit: **minus 5** from negative forces and **plus 3** on positive forces)
- Restrict his business lunches to two per week, with customers only. He will insist that suppliers met him outside lunchtime. On the other three days he will walk to the local delicatessen at lunchtime, buy a sandwich, walk back, and eat at his desk (benefit: **minus 2** from negative forces and **plus 1** on positive forces)
- Drive in his own car to the golf course at weekends so he will be unable to drink alcohol afterwards (benefit: **minus 2** from negative forces)
- Not re-engage his gardener for the imminent spring season. Bob used to enjoy gardening, so he is going to convert some of his lawn into a vegetable plot. This means that he will get plenty of exercise in cultivating it, and it will also make it easier for him to dine healthily on the produce. So, two evenings a week will be spent in the garden rather than

watching TV (benefit: **minus 1** from negative forces and **plus 3** on positive forces)

- Take a different route home from work so that he does not pass his favourite takeaway. Instead, he will stock his refrigerator and freezer with nutritious food than can be cooked quickly and easily as soon as he gets home. He will not keep beer in the house. If he is desperate for a drink on an evening, he will have to make the conscious decision to walk to a local bar or go out and bring back just a few bottles, so that there is no carry over to the next evening (benefit: 4+2 = **minus 6** from negative forces)

Bob decided to make just one of these changes each week over seven weeks. He was confident that this was a goal that he could achieve, whereas he was worried that if he tried to do everything at once he would fail. Any one of these actions in isolation would only have a small effect on his shape, but taken together they resulted in the balance of the Force Field changing to **13:7** in favour of him improving his shape! (**Figure 2.6**).

We can calculate the relative strength of the positive forces using this formula:

$$\% \text{ superiority of positive forces} = ((+ve \text{ forces} - -ve \text{ forces}) \div -ve \text{ forces}) \times 100$$

So,

$$\% \text{ superiority of positive forces} = ((13 - 7) \div 13) \times 100$$
$$= 46\%$$

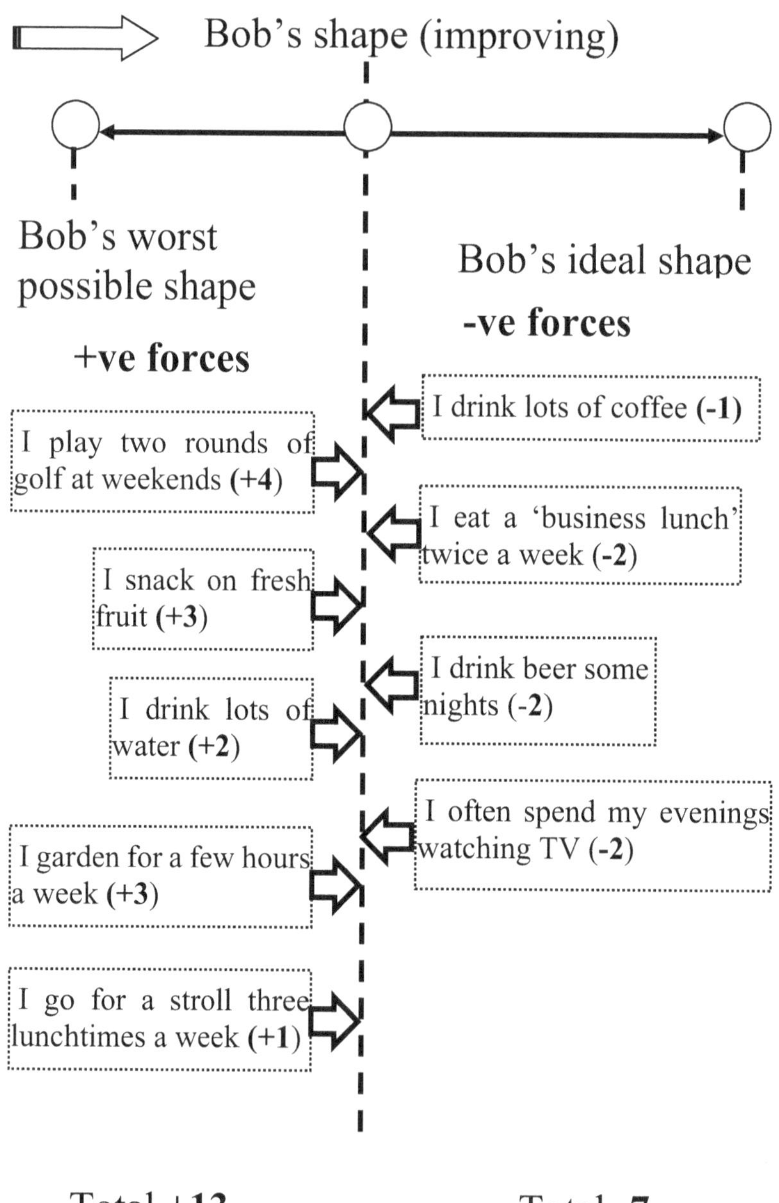

Figure 2.6
Bob's shape (improving)
Bob's worst possible shape
+ve forces
Bob's ideal shape
-ve forces
I drink lots of coffee (-1)
I play two rounds of golf at weekends (+4)
I eat a 'business lunch' twice a week (-2)
I snack on fresh fruit (+3)
I drink beer some nights (-2)
I drink lots of water (+2)
I often spend my evenings watching TV (-2)
I garden for a few hours a week (+3)
I go for a stroll three lunchtimes a week (+1)
Total +13
Total -7

Bob's results

Bob was helped by starting his plan in the spring, rather than in the autumn. He enjoyed walking out to buy a sandwich at lunchtime and cultivating his vegetable plot in the evenings. Other changes were harder, especially giving up drinking bottles of beer every night (or something stronger after playing golf), and dining on junk food. However, Bob succeeded in making these more difficult changes because he had created situations in their favour, by:

- Not keeping beer in the house
- Not being driven home by a friend after playing golf
- Not passing his favourite take-away on the journey home from work

Bob made steady progress toward changing his shape. By the end of the summer, he had shed almost 30 lbs, felt good about himself, and was full of optimism about his career. To continue making progress he was working on a new Force Field diagram for the winter, bringing in regular swimming after work to replace cultivating his garden.

How I used Force Field analysis

When I carried out a Force Field analysis on myself, it showed me that one of the most powerful forces preventing me from improving my shape to the level needed to win bodybuilding competitions was my fondness for a drink on a Saturday night. I was taking in unwanted, empty calories and often felt too lethargic to work up any enthusiasm to go to the gym the next day. If I was going to move my shape up to the next level, I had to find a way to overcome the temptation to drink on a Saturday night. I did this by teaming up with a couple of friends, and arranging to train legs with them at 8am every Sunday morning. My friends were considerably younger and a bit stronger than me, so I knew that they would push me to my limits. We had real 'torture sessions', doing repetition after repetition of deep squats with a 260-pound barbell across our shoulders. The first time we trained, I ended up with a splitting headache from drinking the night before. The experience was so painful that I rarely drank before leg training ever again!

Tips and variations

You should aim for a maximum of ten forces each for or against your shape: if you draw any more than this, then you are probably duplicating some of the forces, or listing irrelevant ones. Although the changes that you make can affect both the positive and negative forces, do not list the absence of a potential negative force as being a positive force: e.g. 'I rarely drink alcohol' is not a positive force, but 'I drink lots of water' is a positive force.

You are going to have to use your intuition to estimate the strength of each force because, as I pointed out in **Chapter 1**, using these tools is sometimes more of an art than a science. However, you do know that, if your shape is deteriorating, then the total score of the negative forces <u>must</u> exceed that of the positive forces (and vice versa if your shape is improving). Also, when weighing up the forces once you have decided what changes to make, do not underestimate the power of a self-fulfilling prophecy. Even if weightings that you have assigned are not quite right, if you believe them, then you will most likely get the results you want.

Once you have designed and implemented a new Force Field, you will need to review it every year or so. One reason for this is that new positive or negative forces may have entered your environment (e.g. the birth of a baby).

The visual impact of the Force Field can be improved by varying the length or thickness of each line according to its strength. If you like, you can draw the opposing forces pulling you into or out of shape, rather than pushing you. Another variation is to draw the continuum vertically rather than horizontally, but I would not recommend this because the forces pushing down the page may then appear to be more powerful because of the perceived effects of gravity.

Alternatively, you could draw the continuum horizontally to represent a seesaw, with the strongest forces for or against your shape being drawn furthest away from the fulcrum and/or being drawn as heavier weights. I have done this for Bob's original and improved Force Fields (**Figures 2.7** and **2.8**, respectively).

The accumulated wisdom, gained from applying Force Field Analysis in a multitude of organizations, is that it is usually more effective to look at altering both the positive and negative forces. This seems to be because, if the positive forces are increased in isolation, then the negative forces tend to strengthen to resist them. Also, as your body moves close to the two extremes of its best or worst possible shape, you will find that the forces pushing it will weaken whilst those restraining it will strengthen, probably because you are pushing against the boundaries set by your genotype. We can draw an analogy here with military supply lines: as they lengthen, they weaken, and as they shorten, they strengthen.

Figure 2.7

Play golf
Drink coffee
Alcohol after golf
Watch TV
Eat takeaways
Snack on chocolate
Skip breakfast
Business lunches
Drink beer
+5 +4 +3 +2 +1 -1 -2 -3 -4 -5
Deterioration

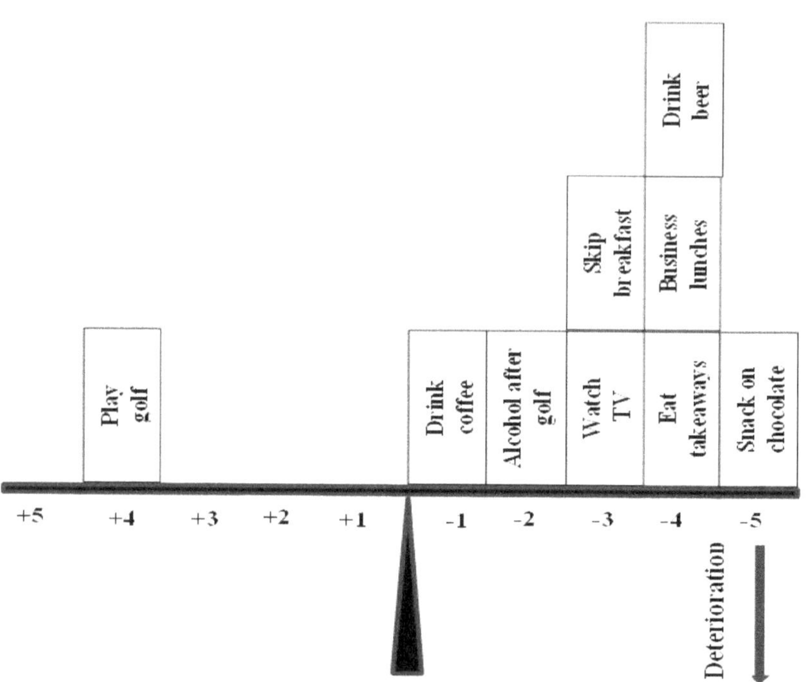

Figure 2.8

Drink beer
Eat fruit
Business lunches
Play golf
Gardening
Drink water
Lunchtime strolls
Drink coffee
Watch TV
+5 +4 +3 +2 +1 -1 -2 -3 -4 -5
Improvement

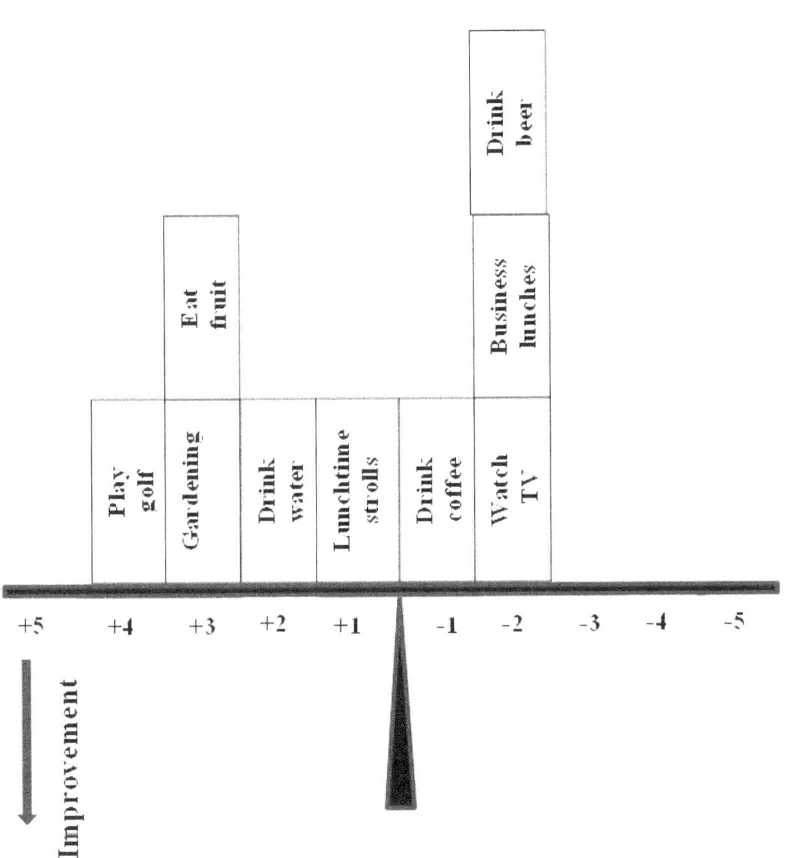

Chapter 3: A new shape by networking (Relationship diagrams)

"Fix the problem, not the blame" (Japanese proverb)

Business background

This chapter features the first of three management tools originating from Japan. In 1972, the Japanese Society of Quality Control Technique Development began to investigate the new tools and techniques that their industries were using to produce goods that were so superior to those of their American and European competitors. They published their findings (in Japanese) in 1979, and the book was translated into English in 1988 as *Management for Quality Improvement: The 7 New QC Tools*, edited by Professor Shigeru Mizumo.

The Relationship diagram is one of these seven new tools: it was being used by the Japanese to clarify, understand, and solve complex problems occurring in their companies. Since then, it has been adopted and used successfully by businesses worldwide.

The basis of the technique is that the factors associated with a problem are spread out on a sheet of paper, and then the relationships between them (in terms of what influences what) are drawn as arrows. Factors with more arrows entering than leaving them are the outcomes or visible symptoms of the problem. Factors with more arrows leaving than entering them are the fundamental causes of the problem: when these are eradicated the problem will be solved.

For example, a Japanese factory was producing too much of its output outside of the very strict tolerances for product quality. Anecdotal evidence suggested that this was because of a poorly trained workforce. However, following a thorough analysis of the problem with a Relationship diagram, the root cause of the problem was found to be the poor layout of machines in the factory. Once this was rectified, product quality improved dramatically.

Key features

Strengths

- This is an excellent tool for identifying the fundamental causes of your current shape
- Use it when the causes of your shape do not fall readily into hierarchical categories, or when there are complex issues surrounding it
- No measuring or data are required
- It is very visual
- There is no need to involve others

But bear in mind

- This is not a tool for monitoring progress towards your new shape
- You need to avoid making the diagram too simple, with arrows pointing in misleading directions; or too complicated, so it is difficult to interpret
- The diagram will need to be redrawn as your circumstances change

The technique explained

You need to begin by defining exactly what the problem is with your current shape. For example:

- I have gained 20 pounds in the last two years
- I can hardly get into any of my clothes
- I am clinically obese
- I am embarrassed to go swimming with my children

Write the problem down on a sticky note. This is your *problem card*.

Next, think about all of the factors in your life that are having a negative effect on your current shape, or that are preventing you from changing it, and jot them down on a sheet of paper. A good start is to take the factors in your Force-Field exercise that you decided were pushing your shape to get worse. However, you <u>must</u> also delve deeper to look for some of the underlying causes, for example:

- I often feel stressed
- I have low willpower
- I am shy

To help you, I have prepared a list of 59 possibilities that you can pick from. Some of these are very similar, some are quite general, and some are very specific, so take your time and choose the most appropriate ones for you. For example, if just one or two of the factors in the list that make up a bad diet apply to you then write them down. However, if several of the factors apply to you then just write that 'my diet is poor'. Notice that under 'attitude' I haven't included the statement that "I don't want to change my shape": the fact that you are reading this book tells me that you do want to change!

Now, by no means is this list meant to be definitive and complete. There are bound to be some factors that apply to you, but that are not on the list, so go ahead and include them. As I pointed out in **Chapter 1**, we are looking for specific solutions to your specific problem, not something that is supposed to work for everyone.

One important point: each factor should contain at least a noun or pronoun, and a verb. Expressions containing a noun alone (e.g. 'children') or a noun and an adjective (e.g. 'inconvenient location') are unlikely to be clear enough. You should aim to identify between 10 and 30 factors that relate to your current situation.

<u>**A list of possible factors**</u>

Diet

- My knowledge of nutrition is poor
- My diet is poor
- I eat lots of sweets and cookies
- I eat lots of fried food
- I eat lots of junk food
- I eat large portions
- I eat when I am not hungry
- I eat lots of takeaways
- I drink lots of sugary drinks
- I don't each much protein
- I often skip meals
- I starve myself then binge
- I eat for comfort
- I eat when I am bored
- I drink beer most nights
- I drink wine with my meals
- I drink too much alcohol
- I drink too much coffee
- I smoke cigarettes
- I don't drink much water
- I start diets then quit
- I don't eat many fruits and vegetables

Exercise

- My knowledge of exercises is poor
- I have no one to exercise with
- None of my friends exercise
- I think that I am using the wrong exercises
- I start to exercise then quit
- I find exercising boring

29

- My gym has poor facilities
- I cannot afford to join a gym
- It takes me a long time to recover between workouts
- I don't exercise much
- I don't exercise very often
- I don't exercise for long
- I don't exercise very intensely
- I don't like people watching me exercise

Attitude

- I don't have much energy to exercise
- I don't have much will-power to diet
- I don't like exercise
- I can't get motivated to diet
- I can't get motivated to exercise
- I often feel stressed
- I am self-conscious of my shape
- All I think about is food
- I am reckless
- I am lazy
- I think that I am too old

Other

- I don't have much time
- My job takes all my time
- My family takes all my time
- My partner takes all my time
- I don't have time to cook
- All my friends are shaped like me
- My partner likes my shape
- All members of my family are shaped like me
- I watch a lot of TV

- I sit down all day at work
- I don't sleep much
- I sleep a lot

Once you feel that you have made a comprehensive list of the factors that are having a bad effect upon your shape, transfer them one-by-one to individual sticky notes, <u>making two sets</u>. These are your *cause cards*. Place one set of cause cards randomly (but evenly) around the perimeter of a sheet of A3 paper (you can make A3 by taping together two sheets of A4). Arranging the cause cards randomly helps to prevent you from making false associations between them. Stick your problem card firmly in the centre of the sheet. Keep the other set of cause cards to one side for use later on. (One simple variation that I will mention here is to use 5" x 3" cards instead of sticky notes and lay these out on a sheet of flip-chart paper).

Now comes the interesting part. Starting at the 12 o'clock position on your sheet, move round the perimeter in a clockwise direction. Each time you come to a cause card, stop, and ask yourself whether or not that factor causes or directly influences either:

- Any of the other factors

And/or

- The central problem itself

If it does, then draw an arrow from that factor to the one(s) that it causes or influences. Think along the lines of *"because of this factor, then the other one happens"*. Move all the way round the cause cards until you end up back at 12 o'clock. Beware of drawing arrows to show weak relationships, because this can result in an important link being obscured by a mass of arrows. Two-way arrows are not allowed: if ever you are tempted to draw one stop and think things through until you are able to 'come of the fence' and identify the most significant direction of influence.

The next step is to take your second set of cause cards and lay them out on another sheet of paper, placing related cards together so that you can draw the arrows linking them without having to leapfrog over several others. It may take you several attempts before you produce your final, tidy version.

Next, on each cause card, write down:

- The number of arrows in (a)
- The number of arrows out (b) (Do not count the arrows going from cause cards to the central problem card)
- The difference between the two (c), where c = a-b. We will call this the *net score*

The card with the biggest <u>negative</u> net score (c) is likely to be the root cause.

Figure 3.1 shows a very simple example that uses just six cause cards. Notice that I have used dashes for the arrows that point to the problem card: this is to remind us that, when we come to count up the arrows, we will not include these. In this example, Cause Card #6 contains the root cause.

Now that you understand the basics, I will describe the application of the technique to a more complex case study.

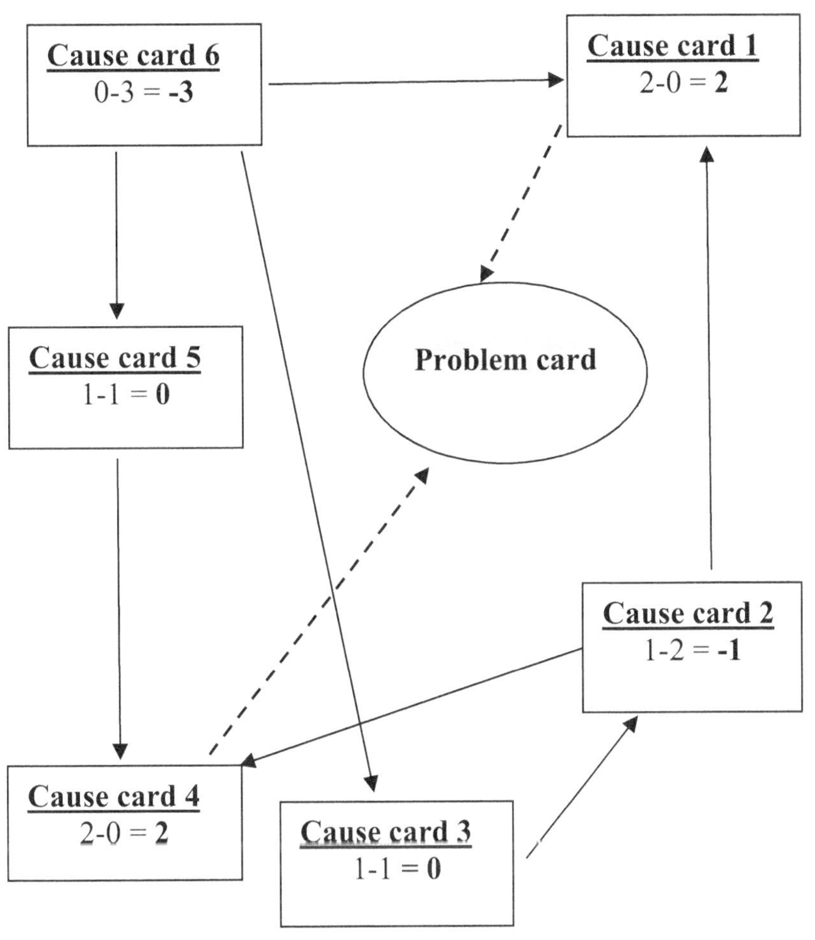

Cause card 6
0-3 = -3
Cause card 1
2-0 = 2
Cause card 5
1-1 = 0
Problem card
Cause card 2
1-2 = -1
Cause card 4
2-0 = 2
Cause card 3
1-1 = 0

Naomi's story

Thirty-five-year-old Naomi is a 'stay at home mum', looking after her three children: Eve (aged two), Tom (seven), and Mark (twelve). Her husband Keith is an advertising executive. He earns good money, but works long hours. Keith was promoted a year ago, but it meant the family moving house to be closer to Head Office and Naomi has struggled to make friends in the new neighbourhood. Consequently, Naomi is lonely during the day.

Looking after her family and home is a very tiring job, especially as she cooks two evening meals, one for her children, and another one later for Keith when he arrives home. Also, because of this, she usually finds herself eating both meals. Being close to the kitchen for most of the day makes it hard for Naomi to resist snacking on cookies.

Before she gave birth to Mark, Naomi had an enjoyable job as college administrator. She would cycle to work, and ate modest amounts of food at normal meal times. In those far-off days she was a size 10, but she is now a size 16. This is her central problem card. Naomi is starting to feel dowdy and unattractive. Keith has also put on weight over the years, but it does not seem to bother him.

Two months ago, Naomi decided to do something to get back into shape. She started one of the 'latest craze' diets, but she failed to stick with it. Although there is a gym close by her home, Naomi felt unable to use it, because she is self-conscious about her poor shape (specifically she did not want to exercise in front of men) and, anyway, she would have had to find someone to look after Eve. Instead, Naomi bought an exercise bike for the spare bedroom. She cycles on it for half an hour whenever Eve has her daytime nap, but she is bored with this routine and wishes she could do something more interesting. Not only that, but she is often so tired that, when Eve has her nap, Naomi joins her on the bed instead of riding the bike.

Naomi's Relationship diagram

Naomi identified 22 factors to put on her cause cards, which she laid out around the central problem of her now being a size 16. After drawing the relationship arrows, she eventually produced the tidied version of her Relationship diagram shown in **Figure 3.2**.

Naomi used a PC, and decided to use a table to record the counts of arrows in and out, so that she could rank the causes by their net scores (see **Figure 3.3**). By doing this, she could see the root causes of her problem (i.e. those with negative net scores) grouped together at the top of the table. These were the things that she had to tackle in order to start dropping dress sizes, and so she decided to:

- Find a facility that has a crèche for Eve and that runs women-only exercise classes during the day. She will aim to attend these on Mondays, Wednesdays, and Fridays, and try to make new, like-minded friends there
- Persuade Keith to join her in getting back into shape. If he agrees, then she will buy a foldaway multi-gym to sit alongside the exercise bike (making sure that it comes with some wall-charts of routines), and she and her husband will work out together on Tuesday and Thursday evenings and at weekends. Mark and Tom can keep an eye on Eve for 45 minutes. Afterwards, they will eat an easily prepared salad or microwave a 'healthy option' type meal from the freezer
- Hire someone to help with the cleaning, washing, and ironing
- Accept that she cannot avoid being close to food for most of the day. However, in order to make her think twice before grazing on high calorie foods throughout the day, she will stick an old photograph of herself in a size 10 dress and an unflattering one of her in a size 16 on the doors of the refrigerator and larder cupboard. She will keep loads of fruit dotted around the house, and will reach for that instead of cookies

- Accept that she could not give up sitting down at the table with her children, but that she would eat, literally, just a saucerful of their meal with them

Naomi's results

Naomi had little difficulty in finding an exercise facility that met her requirements. She really looked forward to the 'step' classes, held on Mondays and Fridays, and the 'spinning' session on Wednesdays. She found that many of the other women there faced problems similar to hers. They were able to help each other to face up to the challenge of improving their shapes. In particular, these new friends were a real source of strength to Naomi in her determination to eat a healthier diet.

Keith was fine about Naomi hiring some domestic help, but he was not keen on making the effort to get into shape himself. Deep down, he just did not believe that this was possible. However, after seeing Naomi drop from a size 16 to a 14 in less than two months, he changed his mind and joined Naomi in working out at home.

Figure 3.2

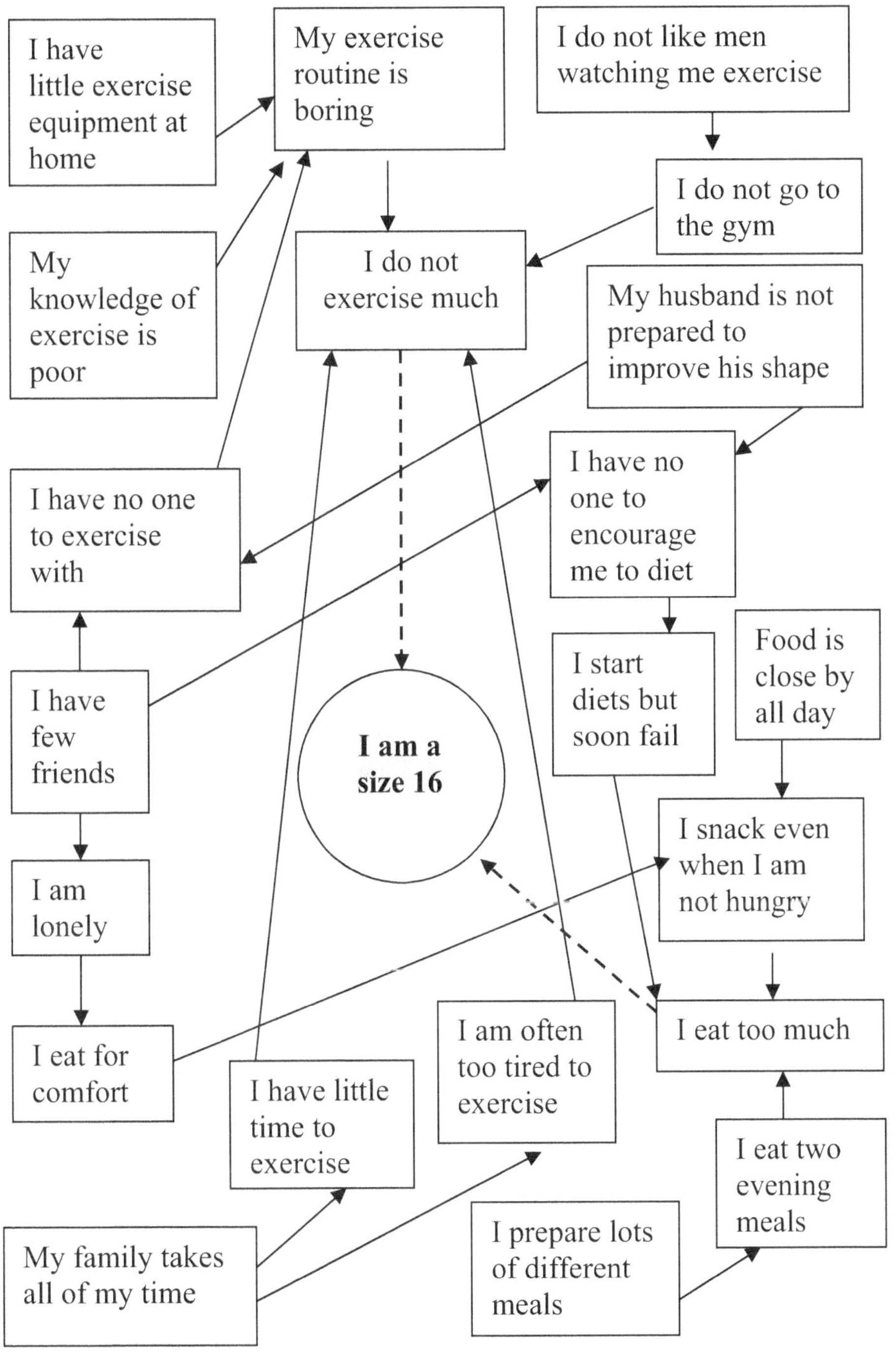

I have little exercise equipment at home
My exercise routine is boring
I do not like men watching me exercise
My knowledge of exercise is poor
I do not exercise much
I do not go to the gym
My husband is not prepared to improve his shape
I have no one to exercise with
I have no one to encourage me to diet
I have few friends
I am a size 16
I start diets but soon fail
Food is close by all day
I am lonely
I snack even when I am not hungry
I eat for comfort
I have little time to exercise
I am often too tired to exercise
I eat too much
My family takes all of my time
I prepare lots of different meals
I eat two evening meals

Figure 3.3

Causes	Arrows in (a)	Arrows out (b)	Net score (c)
I have few friends	0	3	-3
My husband isn't prepared to improve his shape	0	2	-2
My family takes all of my time	0	2	-2
Food is close by all day	0	1	-1
I prepare lots of different meals	0	1	-1
I have little exercise equipment at home	0	1	-1
I do not like men watching me exercise	0	1	-1
My knowledge of exercise is poor	0	1	-1
I am lonely	1	1	0
I start diets but soon fail	1	1	0
I eat for comfort	1	1	0
I eat two evening meals	1	1	0
I have little time to exercise	1	1	0
I do not go to the gym	1	1	0
I am often too tired to exercise	1	1	0
I snack throughout the day even when I am not hungry	2	1	1
I have no one to encourage me to diet	2	1	1
I have no one to exercise with	2	1	1
My exercise routine is boring	3	1	2
I eat too much	3	0*	3
I do not exercise much	4	0*	4

*Remember, we do not count the dashed arrows pointing to the problem card.

How I used a Relationship diagram

In 1998, I was starting to get serious about my bodybuilding, with an eye on competing, but felt that I just wasn't building enough muscle to do so. This was my central problem card. At the time I lived 45 miles away from my job at the University of Sheffield. That meant a 45mile drive to work in a morning, followed by a 45mile drive home. I chose to get home in time to eat with my family at 6.30 pm, which meant that I had to battle through the rush hour traffic to get home from work in time and, after a large meal, I didn't feel like training, especially as I arrived home so stressed out from the drive that I often succumbed to the temptation of a strong drink to unwind. My only opportunity to train during the week was a brief one during my lunch hour, and that just was not enough to build the muscle that I wanted.

After constructing a Relationship diagram **(Figure 3.4)**, the cause of my problem became clear (i.e. always getting back to eat with my family at 6.30), and I solved it by joining the YMCA in Sheffield, and pumping iron there from 5.15 to 6.30 pm on three evenings a week. This enabled me to arrive home calm and relaxed, after a leisurely drive back on quiet roads, and I was able to enjoy my evening meal without a strong drink beforehand.

Tips and variations

When you produce the final, neat version of your Relationship diagram, try arranging the cause cards in a 'directionally intensive' layout, with the problem card at the edge of the page (see **Figure 3.5**).

Alternatively, you can draw different shaped boxes to identify different categories of cause cards e.g. diet, exercise and attitude, or encircle different zones on the Relationship diagram (see **Figure 3.6**). Finally, drawing arrows of varying thickness will help you to indicate the confidence that you have in the relationships and/or the strength of them.

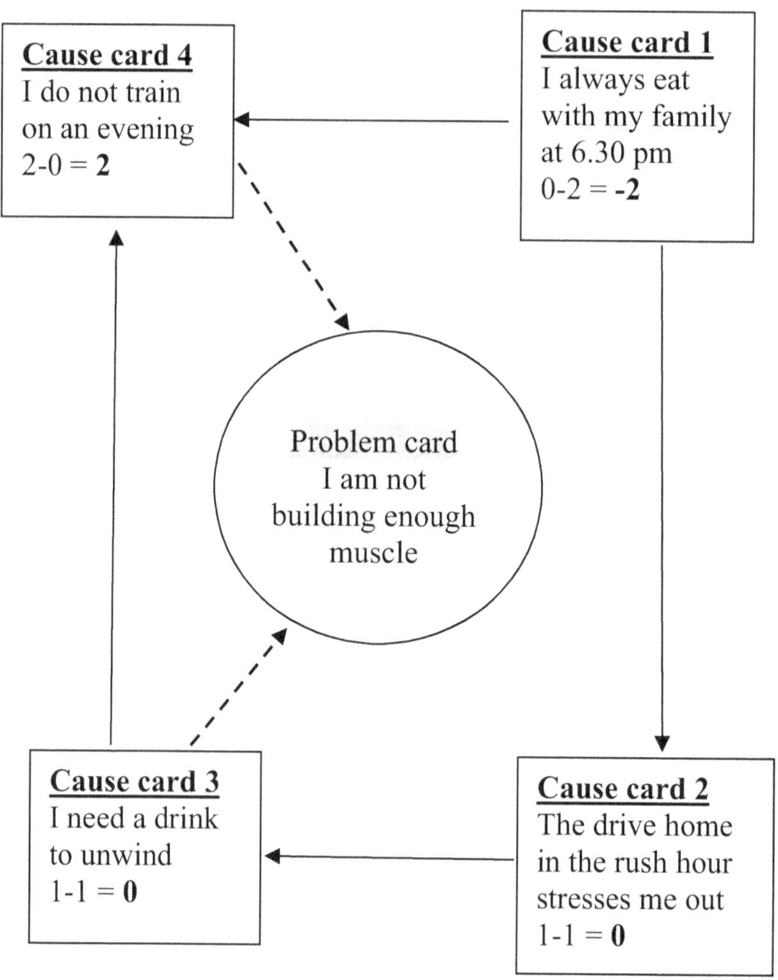
Cause card 4
I do not train
on an evening
2-0 = 2

Cause card 1
I always eat
with my family
at 6.30 pm
0-2 = -2

Problem card
I am not
building enough
muscle

Cause card 3
I need a drink
to unwind
1-1 = 0

Cause card 2
The drive home
in the rush hour
stresses me out
1-1 = 0

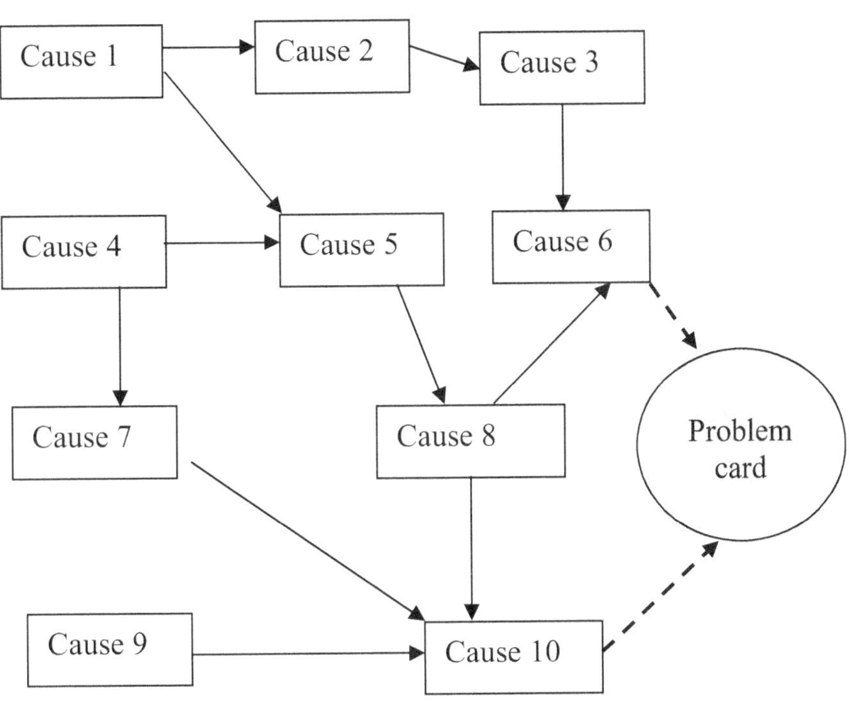

Cause 1
Cause 2
Cause 3
Cause 4
Cause 5
Cause 6
Cause 7
Cause 8
Problem card
Cause 9
Cause 10

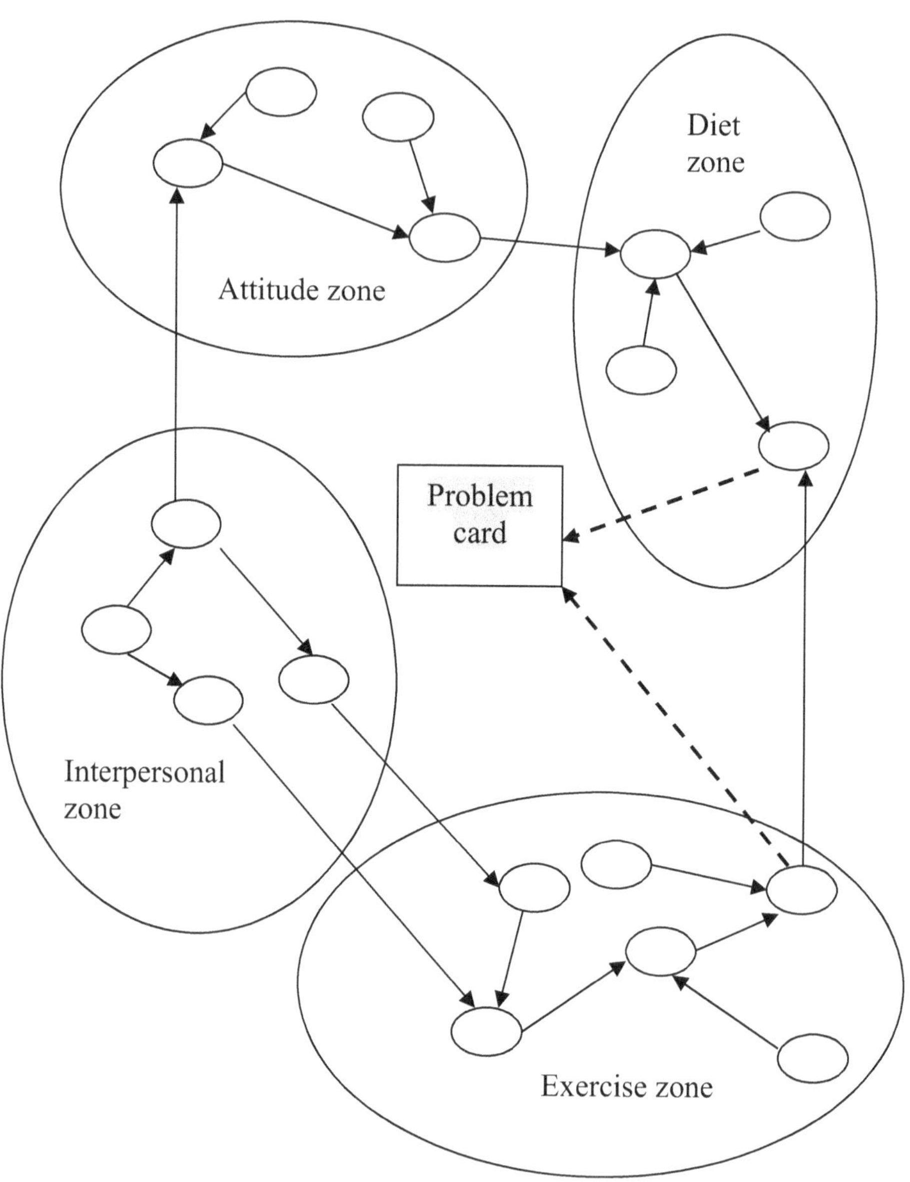

Diet
zone
Attitude zone
Problem
card
Interpersonal
zone
Exercise zone

Chapter 4: Fishing for solutions
(Ishikawa diagrams)

"He who looks outside dreams, he who looks inside wakes" (Carl Jung)

Business background

Kaoru Ishikawa (1915-1989) was a Japanese university professor and key contributor to the development of quality management techniques. He invented the eponymous Ishikawa diagram, and first used it in 1943 at the Kawasaki steel works.

An Ishikawa diagram is a tool with which to discover the major causes of a problem, or the factors governing a task. For example, the automobile manufacturer Mazda used Ishikawa diagrams to help with the design of the hugely successful MX-5 sports car.

The Ishikawa diagram differs from the Relationship diagram that we used in **Chapter 3** by organizing causes into pre-defined categories, instead of scattering them randomly round the perimeter of a sheet of paper. When drawn using angled lines, the resulting pattern resembles the skeleton of a fish: hence the alternative name of Fishbone diagram.

Key features

Strengths

- It will unearth the key causes of your current shape
- Its defined structure helps ensure that all possible causes are recognized
- The hierarchy and frequency of causes are readily identified
- No measuring or data are required
- It is very visual
- There is no need to involve others

- Unlike Force Field and Relationship diagrams, the Ishikawa diagram does not rely on a scoring system

But bear in mind

- The diagram can become so large that it must be split over several sheets of paper
- This is not a tool for monitoring progress towards your new shape
- The diagram will need to be redrawn as your circumstances change

The technique explained

The basic structure of an Ishikawa diagram is shown in **Figure 4.1**. The problem to be solved is written down along the edge of a sheet of paper. Next, a horizontal line and four diagonals are drawn. These diagonals are the *cause areas*. Lines are drawn to represent different *aspects* of the cause areas. Within each aspect, the specific *causes* of the problem are identified, and can then be dealt with.

It may be that you can identify, and then deal with, a cause that is linked directly to an aspect. However, it is more likely that a cause will lead you to a *sub-cause*, and perhaps then on to a *sub-sub-cause* etc. To solve your problem, you need to deal with those causes/sub-causes/sub-sub-causes that have no other lines leading from them. I have shown these in bold in **Figure 4.2**.

If we were to use the Ishikawa diagram to diagnose a problem in a business then we might label the cause areas:

- Manpower, Machines, Methods, and Materials

Or

- Place, Procedure, People and Policies

Or

- Surroundings, Suppliers, Systems and Skills

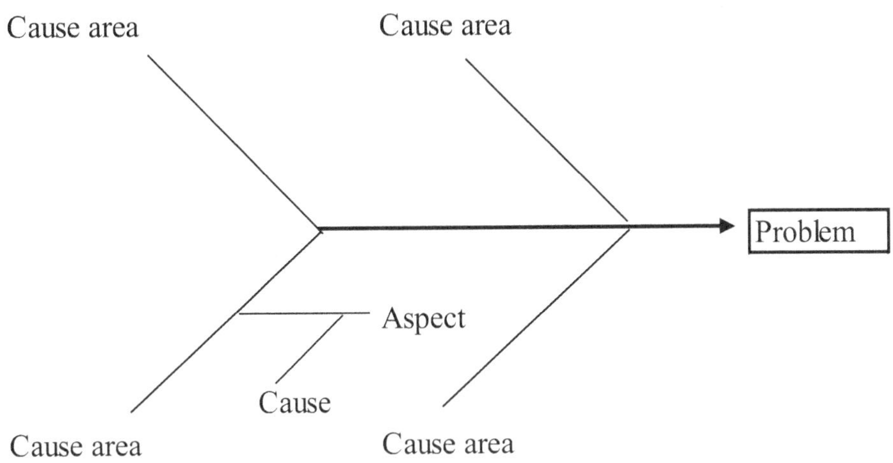

Figure 4.1

Figure 4.2

Innovatively, for our purpose, we will label them Diet, Exercise, Rest and Mind. We now need to decide what aspects to use within each of these four cause areas. For Diet, Exercise and Rest, the causes will fall within the aspects of: Quantity, Quality, and Pattern, whilst for Mind, the aspects are: Knowledge, Attitude and Habits. I have constructed an Ishikawa diagram using these labels in **Figure 4.3**. This is our basic template.

Just as in **Chapter 3**, the first step is for you to state precisely what is wrong with your current shape. Be specific and do not pull any punches. Let's assume you decide that the problem is 'My belly hangs over my belt'. You now need to consider what the causes of that problem are within each of the 12 aspects. For example, you might decide that a contributory factor to your belly hanging over your belt, within the aspect *Quality of Exercise,* is that you do not train your abdominal muscles. Ask yourself:

Question - *Why do I not train my abdominal muscles?*
Answer - *Because it hurts my back*

And then:

Question - *Why does it hurt my back?*
Answer – *Because the sit-up bench has very thin padding*

Add these to the Ishikawa diagram as in **Figure 4.4**. Keep on going until you have isolated the 'end' causes for each of the aspects, and then decide what you are going to do to tackle these causes. Possible solutions to the end cause in **Figure 4.4** would be to buy a new sit-up bench that has thick padding, or join a gym that is equipped with such an item.

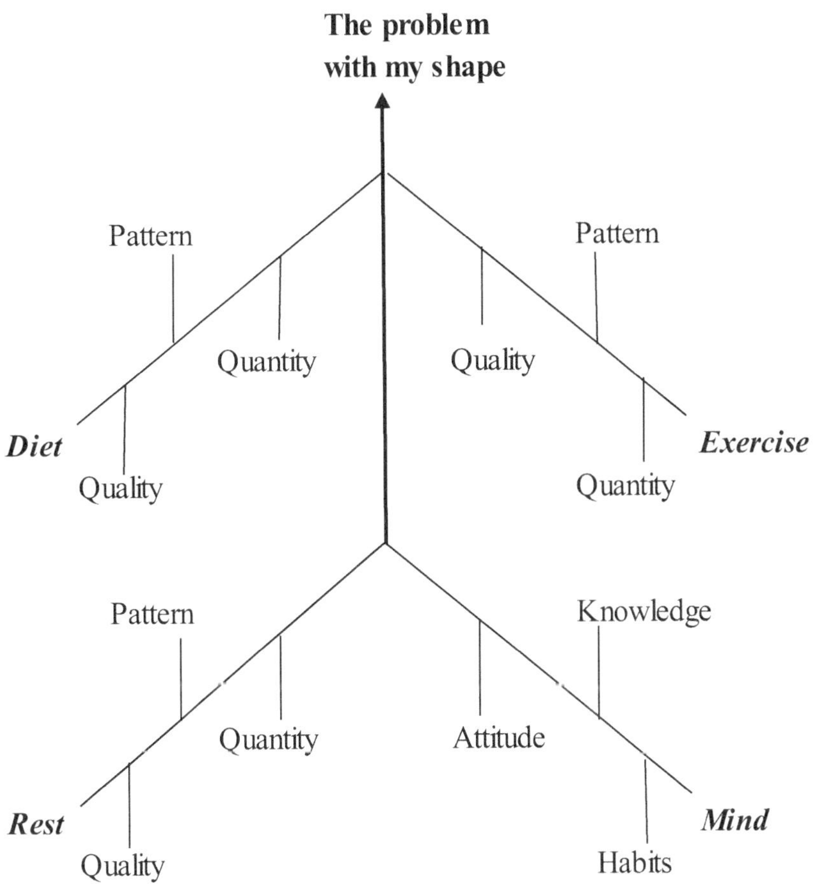
The problem
with my shape
Pattern
Pattern
Quantity
Quality
Diet
Quality
Exercise
Quantity
Pattern
Knowledge
Quantity
Attitude
Rest
Mind
Quality
Habits

<u>Figure 4.4</u>

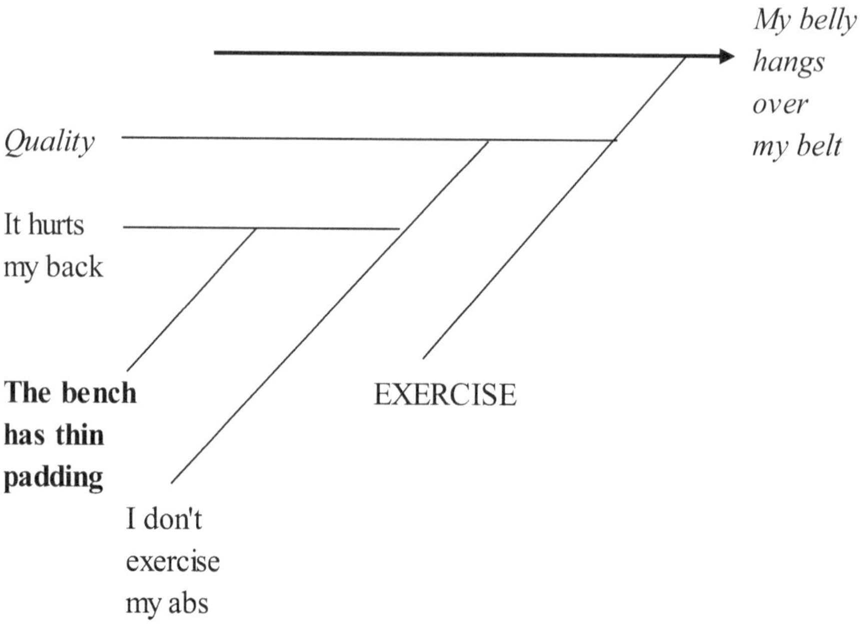

The compendium of causes that you identify will be unique to your problem, your body, and your lifestyle. Remember, something <u>must</u> be causing the problem; otherwise the problem would not exist. To help you to isolate the cause(s), I have listed below the sorts of things you should consider:

<u>Diet</u>

Quantity

- Calorific value
- Portion size
- Water intake

Quality

- Nutrient profile (protein, carbohydrate, fat)

- Fruit and vegetable intake
- Fibre intake
- Glycaemic index
- Supplementation with vitamins etc.
- Salt intake
- Caffeine intake
- Alcohol intake[1]

Pattern

- Frequency[2]
- Regularity[3]
- Skipping breakfast
- Eating late at night

Exercise

Quantity

- Hours per week spent exercising
- Distance ran, swam, walked, or cycled
- Number of reps in the gym
- Total kg lifted in the gym

Quality

- Intensity
- Variety
- Correct form
- Appropriateness

Pattern

- Frequency[2]
- Regularity[3]

<u>Rest</u>

Quantity

- Hours of sleep per week

Quality

- Partner snoring
- Crying baby
- Noisy neighbours
- Jet lag
- Shift work
- Alcohol intake[1]
- Stress

Pattern

- Frequency[2]
- Regularity[3]

<u>Mind</u>

Knowledge

- Of nutrition
- Of exercise

Attitude

- Motivation
- Willpower
- Positivity/negativity
- Peer pressure/support
- Self-esteem

50

- Prioritisation
- Willingness to do new things

Habits

- Procrastination
- Smoking
- Drinking alcohol[1]
- Watching television

1. Some causes (e.g. alcohol intake) will occur in more than one cause area.

2. Frequency = the length of intervals between events.

3. Regularity = the degree to which events occur at the same time each day, or each week.

We will now move on to our case study to see the Ishikawa diagram in action.

Emily's story

By most standards, Emily has done very well in her 32 years of life. Intelligent, industrious, and personable, she graduated with a first-class degree, and represented her university at hockey and swimming, before landing a job with a leading law firm. Single and childless herself, she specializes in divorce law, and is willing to represent clients of either sex in their quest for an equitable end to a failed marriage.

Emily gives 100 percent commitment and effort to her job. She works at a frenetic pace all day long, and often brings casework home to read. Actually, just about the only time Emily is at home during the week (apart from sleeping) is when she reads through her casework. She finds it depressing to cook and eat on her own, so she dines out with friends on most nights during the week.

On Saturdays, Emily trawls the shops and boutiques for clothes and other items that she does not really need, and then she either hosts a dinner party or attends one elsewhere. On Sundays, she lays in bed until late, does her domestic chores and then visits her parents. Nevertheless, Emily does manage to fit in a three-mile jog on both Saturdays and Sundays.

Emily rises early for work. Breakfast is usually a bowl of muesli, followed by a sandwich for lunch. She snacks on fruit during the day.

Recently, Emily has started to notice changes in the shape of her body. Almost imperceptible at first, there is now no doubt that her bottom is getting bigger, her limbs are getting flabbier and her once taut tummy is getting softer. Although Emily would not be classed as overweight in comparison to the majority of the population, she is no longer the proud owner of an athletic body.

Emily's reaction to this was two-fold: she cut down on her food intake by skipping either breakfast or lunch on alternate weekdays, and extended her jogging route by an extra mile. Unfortunately, this did not restore her shape.

Alarmed by this, and worried by the certainty that her shape would undoubtedly deteriorate further unless she took the appropriate action, Emily decided to draw an Ishikawa diagram to identify the causes of her worsening shape.

Emily's Ishikawa diagram

Emily began by stating her problem as '*I no longer have an athletic body*'. She then brainstormed the possible reasons for this under each aspect, scribbling them down on a sheet of paper before selecting the ones with which to construct her Ishikawa diagram.

Diet (Figure 4.5)

After reviewing her diet, Emily calculated that the quantity of food she was consuming was about right at c.2000 Kilocalories a day.

However, she acknowledged that the pattern of consumption was not good, with intake occurring mainly on an evening. This was partly due to her habit of dining in restaurants or at parties: this also accounted for a negative factor within the quality of her diet, in that it contained significant amounts of alcohol. After asking herself why this was she concluded, somewhat reluctantly, that the underlying cause was that she was lonely and wanted companionship.

Figure 4.5

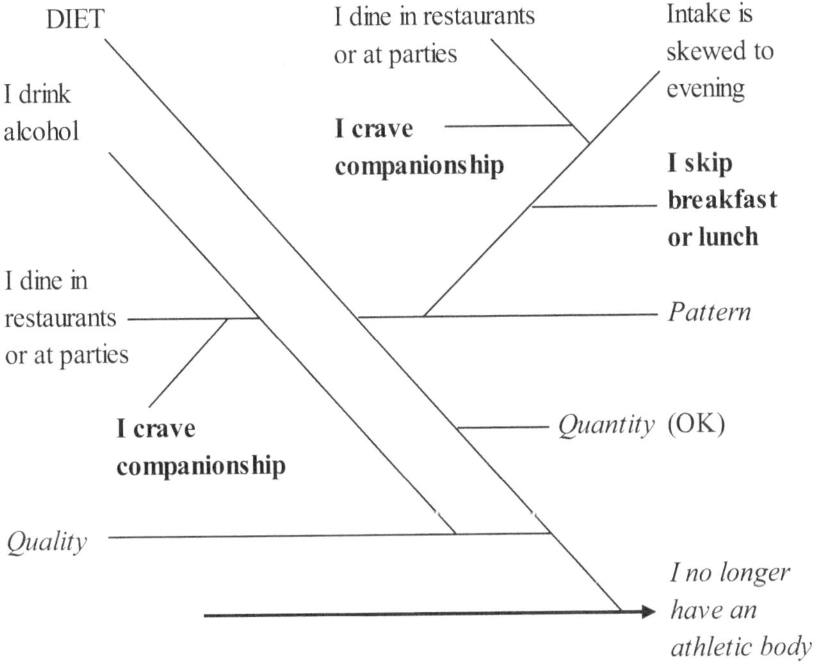

Exercise (Figure 4.6)

Emily decided that, because she was running eight miles a week, the quantity of exercise that she was subjecting her body to was OK. Having said that, jogging was the only exercise she did, and she only did it at weekends. This was because she had no facilities for any other type of exercise, and because her work and need to socialize took priority during the week.

Figure 4.6

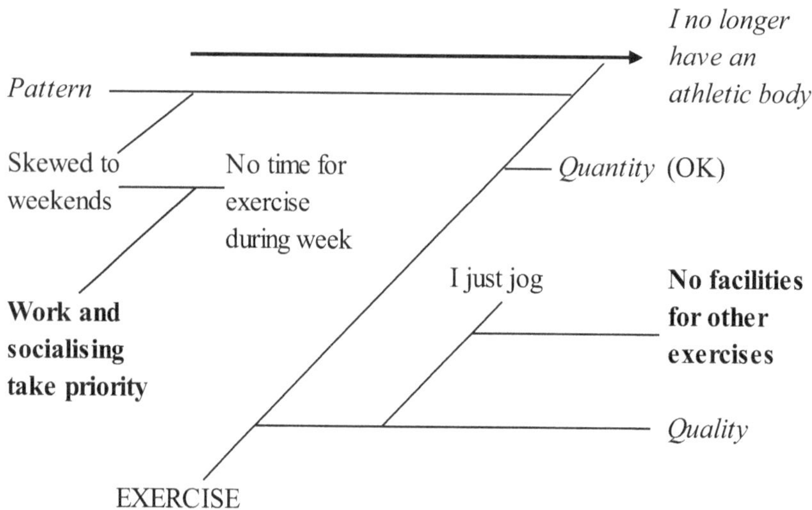

Rest (Figure 4.7)

Just as there was no overt problem with the quantity of food consumed, or exercise undertaken, Emily worked out how much sleep she got a week and decided that at c.54 hours a week she was doing fine. But, once again, there were issues with the pattern and quality of her sleep that needed to be addressed. Emily was barely sleeping seven hours a night during the week, compared to ten hours a night at weekends, and her sleep was often interrupted by periods of wakefulness. Her Ishikawa diagram enabled her to identify the ubiquitous, underlying causes of: a craving for companionship; and the priority that she gave to work and socializing.

Figure 4.7

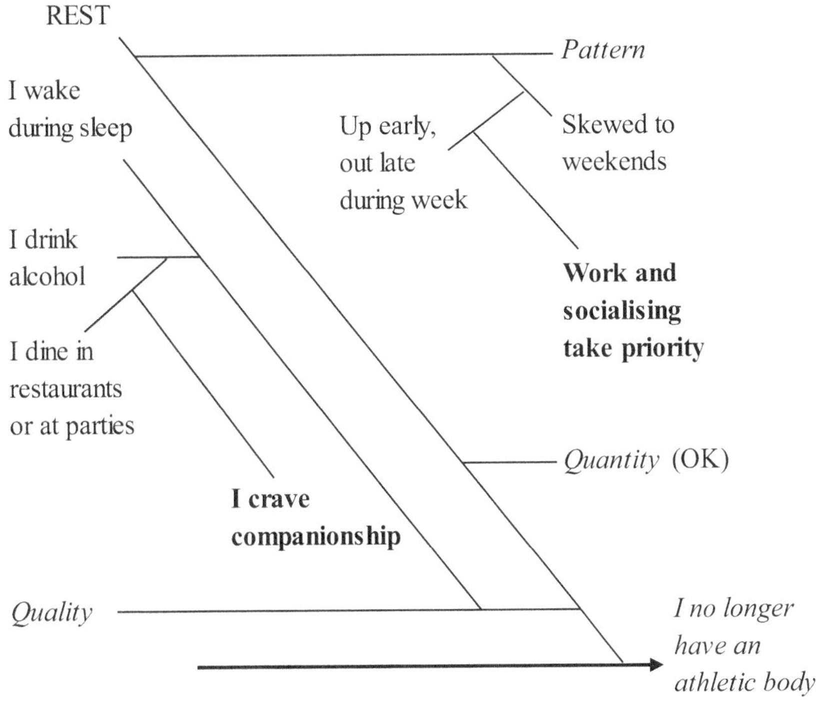

Mind (Figure 4.8)

Emily identified the underlying causes of her problem that were attached to all three aspects of the Mind cause area. Two new causes emerged: Emily had little knowledge of structured training; and none of her friends were trying to improve their own shapes.

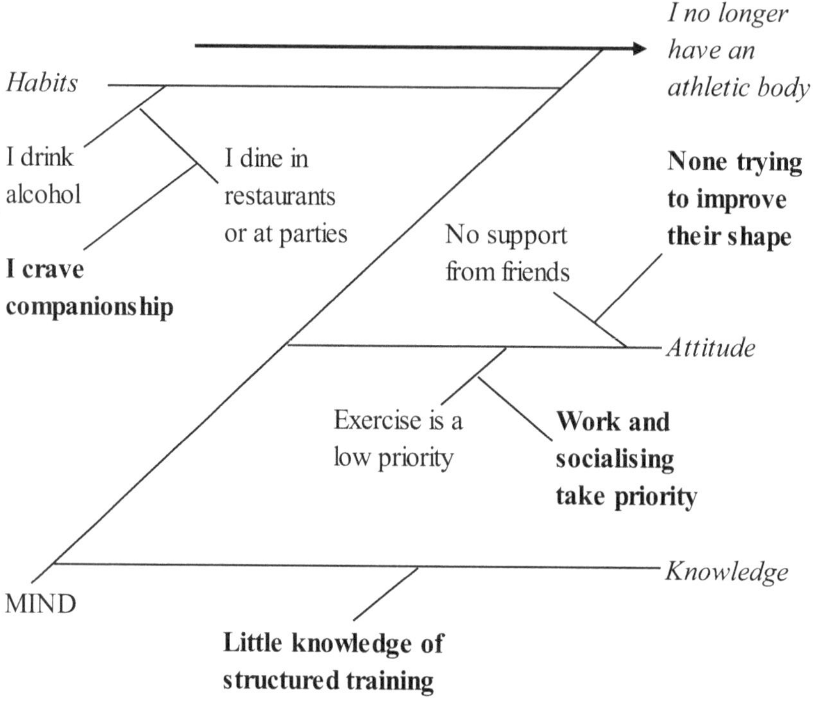

Action taken

Emily listed the underlying causes from her Ishikawa diagram. In order of the number of occurrences, these were:

- I crave companionship (4 occurrences)
- Work and socializing take priority (3 occurrences)
- None of my friends are trying to improve their shape (1 occurrence)
- I have no facilities for other exercises (1 occurrence)
- I have little knowledge of structured training (1 occurrence)
- I skip breakfast or lunch (1 occurrence)

The last of these causes was easily rectified: Emily reverted to eating a bowl of muesli topped with fruit for breakfast and a variety of sandwiches at lunchtime each day. The solution to overcoming the remaining causes virtually 'flew out of the page' at her. What she needed to do was to find a way of combining socializing with exercising.

She contemplated joining a swimming or running club but, instead, she joined her local orienteering club (orienteering is a sport in which the participant navigates their way round an unmarked course, often in a forest, using a map and compass). Events were held on most Sundays, with classes of varying difficulty to cater for participants of all abilities. Emily wanted to do her best in this new sport, so she began to watch the amount she drank the Saturday night before. Members of the club shared lifts in cars, or hired a bus to events, so there was plenty of opportunity to talk and to get to know each other.

Next, she visited her nearest leisure centre to enquire about what she could do there on weekday evenings. After talking to the staff on the front desk, she decided to try the badminton sessions that were held every Wednesday evening. Around twenty people joined Emily for her first session, and with just three badminton courts available, this meant that Emily was compelled to play doubles with a variety of partners. She was pleased to find that she knew two of the players from the orienteering club. These two women were focused on keeping fit, so they worked out in the adjacent gym on Mondays and Thursdays. Emily asked if she could join them, and soon they became her good friends.

Prior to exercising on weekday evenings, Emily ate a simple meal, at her desk, of something like a baked potato with cheese and salad, washed down with water, not wine. She still joined her old friends for a restaurant meal on the remaining evenings but, to be honest, she no longer enjoyed these occasions very much because of the air of negativity and recklessness surrounding them.

Emily's results

Emily's previous pattern of eating very little during the day, and a lot at night, had caused her to gain unwanted fat. Her body had reacted to this regime by setting its metabolism to a very low level during the day and then storing the glut of night-time nutrients as fat. The switch to eating during the day, combined with exercising on an evening, accelerated Emily's metabolic rate so that she began to shed fat.

The introduction of resistance exercises into her regime improved the strength, tone, and shape of Emily's muscles, so that she no longer had flabby limbs.

The changes that Emily made to her lifestyle in order to get these results were not difficult or uncomfortable: far from it. Emily felt good about herself; she had a lot more energy and had several new, like-minded friends.

How I used an Ishikawa diagram

My early attempts to transform my physique in 1995 were unsuccessful. Although I was lifting heavy weights in the gym, I just was not adding muscle like I expected. I constructed an Ishikawa diagram to help me understand why this was. The chain of events was that: I was not growing because I was not eating enough - because I often had no appetite - because I smoked a pipe (**Figure 4.9**). So, apart from any other bad effects that smoking tobacco was having on my body, I had to quit if I was serious about getting a muscular body.

Now, those of you who have tried to quit smoking will know just how difficult it is. I soon discovered that my desire to add muscle was not strong enough to overcome my cravings for a pipeful of tobacco, so I had to find another motivator. What I did was to use mental imagery to visualize myself in hospital dying from lung cancer, surrounded by my four children, knowing that I would never see them grow up. The emotions attached to this awful scenario were so powerful that they conquered my cravings for nicotine.

<u>Figure 4.9</u>

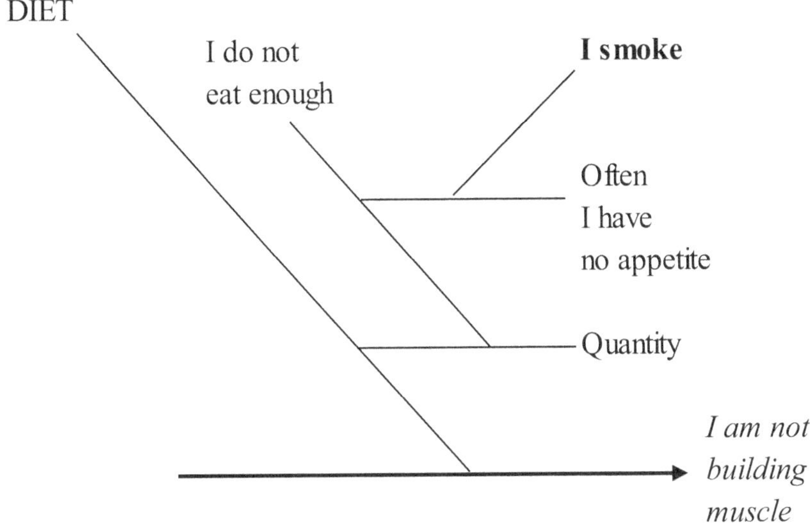

Tips and variations

Using angled lines for the diagrams should allow you to fit more lines on a page, but you can draw the diagrams using a right-angled grid (**Figures 4.10** and **4.11** are modifications of **Figures 4.1** and **4.2**, respectively). Either way, you will probably find it easier to draw your diagram on four sheets of paper, one for each cause area.

I reiterate that you are unique, and that these tools will produce solutions that are specific to you and your situation. So, you will find that some cause areas and aspects will be more appropriate to you than others, but be wary of areas of your Ishikawa diagram with no attached causes at all. Make sure that you have thought things through, and that you are being completely honest with yourself.

59

Cause area
Cause area
Problem
Aspect
Cause
Cause area
Cause area

Figure 4.11

Problem
Cause
Aspect
Sub-cause
Aspect
Cause
Sub-cause
Sub-sub-cause
Cause
Cause area

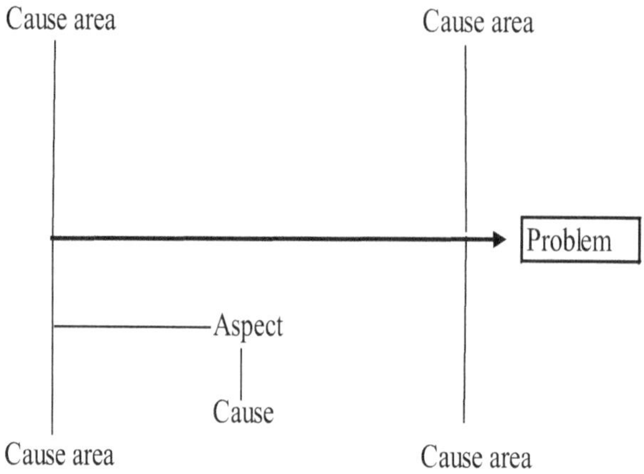

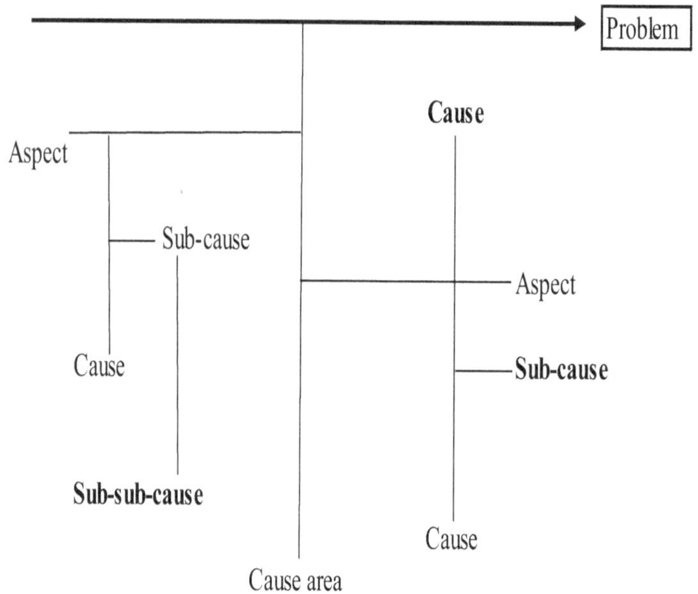

Although I have shown how Emily ranked the importance of causes by counting the frequency of their occurrence, the Ishikawa diagram does not rely on a scoring system. However, you can bring more arithmetic into your diagram by scoring the degree of confidence that you have in each of the underlying causes that you identify:

- If your basis for identifying an underlying cause is just based on a hunch, then give it a score of 1
- If you have a lot of confidence in the validity of the cause, then score it 3
- Give anything in between a score of 2

You can then work out which are the major causes to act on by using the following formula:

Importance of cause = Number of occurrences × Confidence score

Chapter 5: Getting to the root of things (Tree diagrams)

"It is never too late to be what you might have been"
(Mary Ann Evans)

Business background

The Tree diagram is the third (and final) management tool originating from Japan to be featured in this book. In common with the Relationship diagram, which we used in **Chapter 3**, it appeared in the 1988 book *Management for Quality Improvement: The 7 New QC Tools*, in which it was described as the *Systemic* diagram. Sometimes, it is also referred to as a *Dendrogram*.

In that book, the late Professor Shigeru Mizumo describes how the technique was used by the television industry in Japan to produce a high-quality, low-cost receiver.

Key features

Strengths

- This tool will give you a clear picture of the route that will take you from your current shape to your desired shape
- This is a very positive, motivational technique
- It is logical and systematic
- No measuring or data are required
- There is no need to involve others

But bear in mind

- You will probably get through a lot of pencil lead and paper before you produce your finished version!
- Because there are no pre-defined categories, it is possible for you to overlook some of the steps that you need to take

- It is unlikely that the diagram will fit on a sheet of A4: you will probably need to use A5

The technique explained

An objective is defined, beneath which the ways and means to achieve it are stated. These ways and means then become sub-objectives, to which are attached a further level of ways and means. The process is repeated until a clear path from the current state to the ultimate objective appears. The finished diagram resembles the root system or branches of a tree. A similar layout is also used in organizational charts and family trees, so you should already be familiar with it.

Begin by visualizing the shape that you want. Be ambitious, but be realistic: think about a shape that you believe is attainable within a year or two. You need to have a crisp, clear picture of this, your new shape; because you must then go one stage further and believe that you already have it! This is why the Tree diagram is such an excellent motivational tool: you work back from this ideal shape, instead of starting out with your current shape.

Write down the fact that you have this new shape, and then start to think about how you got it, asking yourself '*How did that happen?*' Start by answering this question with a high-level statement e.g. '*I lost fat and gained muscle*' and keep on repeating the process, drilling down until you arrive at a set of answers that are specific, discrete and, above all, readily actionable. Here is an example in **Figure 5.1**.

Figure 5.1 assumes that, in order to lose fat and gain muscle, you exercised more and ate properly: so these two ways and means are written at the next level down. In order to exercise more you did several different things and, similarly, various actions contributed to you eating properly. One of these latter actions was that you stopped eating chocolate. You were able to stop eating chocolate because, amongst other things, you started to associate chocolate with fat.

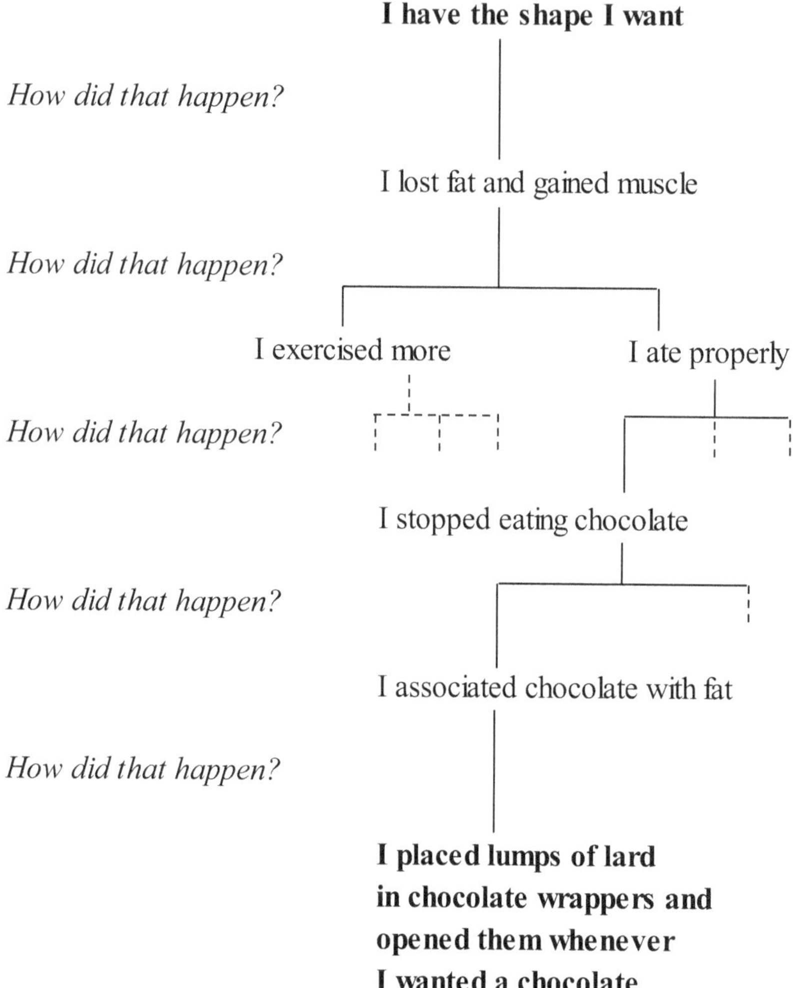

In turn, this came about because you placed lumps of lard inside chocolate wrappers, which you opened whenever you felt the urge to eat chocolate. This is your final <u>actionable</u> statement: doing it today will start the sequence of events that culminate in your shape being the one that you want.

Amber's story

Amber has been overweight for as long as she can remember. Equipped with big bones and big hips, just like her mother and sister, at 26 years old she now weighs 175 pounds at a height of 5 feet 8 inches.

She has become well and truly accustomed to being described as 'plump' or 'chubby'. Although she acts as though this does not bother her, underneath the façade she is hurting. She dreams of dating and maybe settling down with a handsome man, but she feels so unattractive, and has so little self-esteem, that she just cannot see it ever happening with her current shape.

Amber works as a personal assistant to a director of a large insurance company. She drives to work, where she more or less sits at her desk all day long. Her only forms of exercise are doing the housework and walking the aisles of her local supermarket.

Amber eats what she would describe as a 'normal' sort of diet. Breakfast is a hurried couple of slices of toast, lunch is a meal in her employer's on-site canteen, and dinner is something micro-waved from the freezer. In between, she snacks on cookies and chocolate bars, but not excessively. She is not a big drinker: her intake of alcohol is usually confined to Saturday nights when she goes out 'clubbing' with her girlfriends.

Every now and again, Amber will try one of the latest 'fad' diets. Full of hope, and brimming with enthusiasm, she will follow the diet and lose several pounds in the first fortnight. However, she will then invariably find the diet unbearable and quit it, quickly regaining the weight that she had worked so hard to shed.

She has almost resigned herself to staying frustrated, bitter, and unhappy inside her unattractive shape for the rest of her life but, before she finally gives up, Amber has decided to see if using a Tree diagram will enable her to get the shape that she wants.

Amber's Tree diagram

This is shown in **Figure 5.2**. At the outset, Amber spent some time visualizing her new, sexy, feminine body. She then stated that she already had this body at the top of a sheet of paper. This initial statement was in the present tense: all subsequent statements would be in the past tense, as if they had already happened. Amber reasoned that three things had happened for her to get this body: she believed that it was possible; she had a good diet; and she exercised properly. These were written at the next level down.

Despite all her previous negative attitudes, Amber was able to believe that her new shape could happen. This was because she spent a set amount of time each week in reading motivational literature, and in reinforcing the shape of her new body in her mind by visualization.

Amber's diet was good: not only had she spent several hours a week (at the outset) in learning about nutrition and the importance of body types before choosing an appropriate diet, she had also managed to stick to her diet. Three factors enabled Amber to keep to her diet:

- The diet was sustainable, because it was designed to result in a weight loss of just 1lb a week. Amber monitored and controlled her new diet to this end by weighing herself every Saturday morning, and by keeping a daily diary of her food intake
- Every Sunday, Amber planned her menus for the week ahead. She bought the ingredients and did as much preparatory work as possible
- She joined a good health club so that she could receive support from others who had also decided to eat a planned diet

Amber added each of these steps to her Tree diagram before turning her attention to thinking about what had resulted in her exercising properly. She decided that this had happened because:

- She had the facilities to exercise (by joining a good health club)
- She knew what exercises to do (by hiring a personal trainer)
- She actually did the exercises (by training for an hour a day, six days a week)

These were the final additions to the Tree diagram. Amber reviewed the finished diagram, and saw that there were just eight things that she needed to do in order to start the chain of events that would lead to her having a sexy, feminine body in the flesh, not just in her mind's eye.

I have shown these eight actions in italics in **Figure 5.2**. Joining a health club and hiring a personal trainer were one-off actions by Amber. Reading information on nutrition and body types was something to be done just for the first few weeks. The remaining five actions were on-going.

Amber's results

Amber realized that her inherited characteristics would make it difficult for her to acquire a lean, athletic physique, so she visualized herself having a voluptuous, curvy, feminine body. In fact, each night as she lay in bed before drifting off to sleep, Amber focused on an image of her face on the body of Marilyn Monroe!

Amber was able to keep to her diet with ease, simply because it was nowhere near as difficult as some of the crash diets that she had attempted in the past. However, exercising six times a week was much more challenging, mainly because this was something that Amber had never done before. The key success factors here were the guidance that she obtained from her personal trainer, together with the encouragement that she received from the staff and other members of the health club.

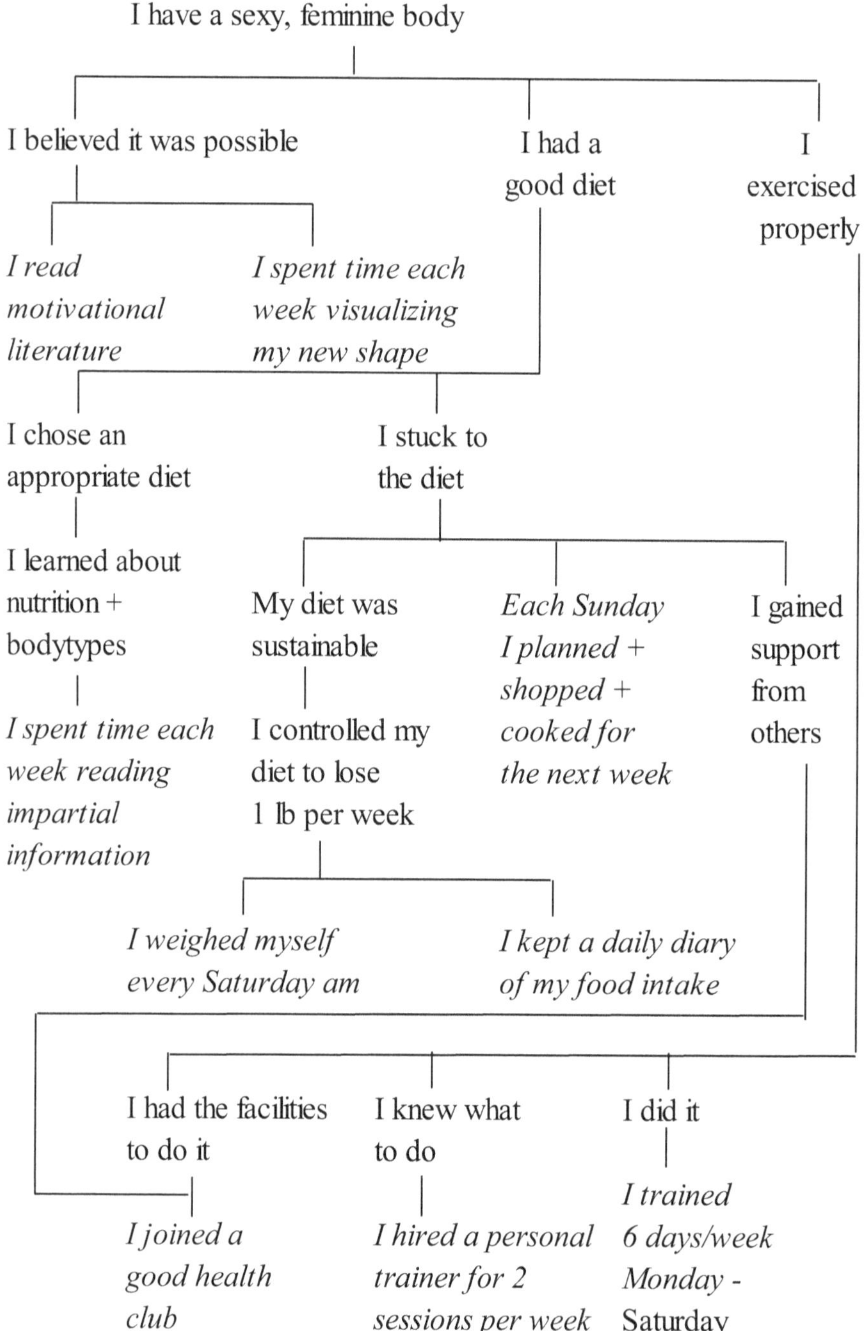

I have a sexy, feminine body
I believed it was possible
I had a good diet
I exercised properly
I read motivational literature
I spent time each week visualizing my new shape
I chose an appropriate diet
I stuck to the diet
I learned about nutrition + bodytypes
I spent time each week reading impartial information
My diet was sustainable
I controlled my diet to lose 1 lb per week
Each Sunday I planned + shopped + cooked for the next week
I gained support from others
I weighed myself every Saturday am
I kept a daily diary of my food intake
I had the facilities to do it
I knew what to do
I did it
I joined a good health club
I hired a personal trainer for 2 sessions per week
I trained 6 days/week Monday - Saturday

Figure 5.2

<u>Figure 5.3</u>

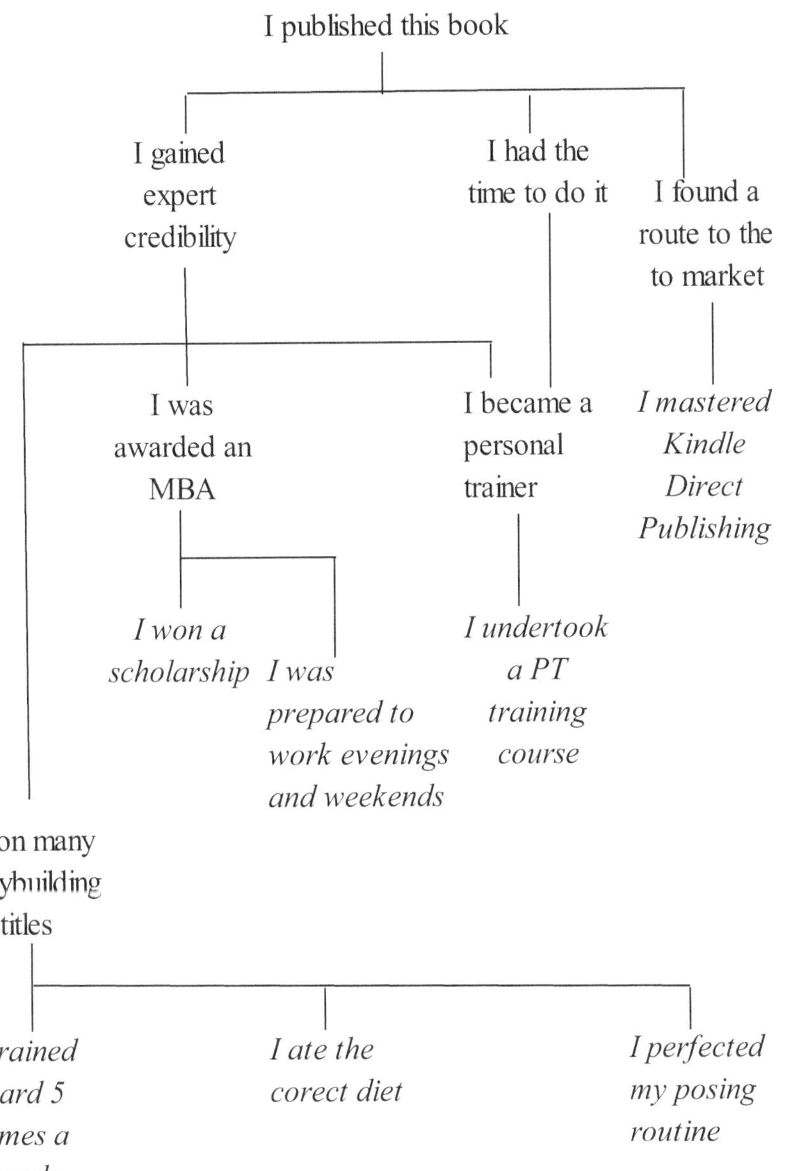
I published this book
I gained expert credibility
I had the time to do it
I found a route to the to market
I was awarded an MBA
I became a personal trainer
I mastered Kindle Direct Publishing
I won a scholarship
I was prepared to work evenings and weekends
I undertook a PT training course
I won many bodybuilding titles
I trained hard 5 times a week
I ate the corect diet
I perfected my posing routine

The shape of Amber's body began to change, albeit slowly. This gave Amber the confidence to believe that her Tree diagram was working, and the extra motivation to stick to it, motivation that was increased dramatically whenever she noticed guys gazing at her. Although she never quite achieved the shape of Marilyn Monroe, her new body, and especially the confidence that came with it, enabled her to date the type of man that she had always dreamt of.

How I used a Tree diagram

I used this technique to develop and implement a plan to become a successful author (**Figure 5.3**). This was a long-term plan, so the seven key actions were not all scheduled to occur simultaneously.

Tips and variations

You may find it easier to construct your Tree diagram if you locate your initial statement in the centre of the page (**Figure 5.4**) or the top left-hand corner (**Figure 5.5**).

Whatever layout you decide upon, you should check on the logic within it before implementing it. The way to do this is to make sure that, when you read it in reverse order (i.e. from the lowest levels to the highest one), you can explain the links by the statement *"this allowed me to"*.

Make sure that you look at your root actions and decide: which of them are one-offs, which of them are transient and which of them are continuous. Think through, and decide upon the order in which you are going to implement them, before actually going ahead with them.

You can construct your Tree diagram to look backwards, so as to analyze the reasons for your current shape. Although I do not find this as motivational as looking forward to the body you want, this is how to do it:

- Start with a statement that describes your current shape (e.g., 'I am three stone overweight')
- At the next level down, give the direct causes of this (e.g., 'I eat a lot of puddings')
- Keep on drilling down as before until you find the root causes that you can take action to eradicate. For example, maybe you eat a lot of puddings because your partner always cooks dinner and includes a dessert that you find hard to resist. You can partially solve this by taking it in turns to cook dinner and omitting the dessert course when it is your turn to cook

Figure 5.4

Level 5
Level 5
Level 4
Level 4
Level 3
Level 3
Level 3
Level 4
Level 3
Level 2
Level 2
Level 4
Level 1
I have the body I want
Level 1
Level 1
Level 2
Level 2
Level 2
Level 3
Level 3
Level 2
Level 3
Level 4
Level 3
Level 3
Level 4
Level 4
Level 4
Level 5
Level 5

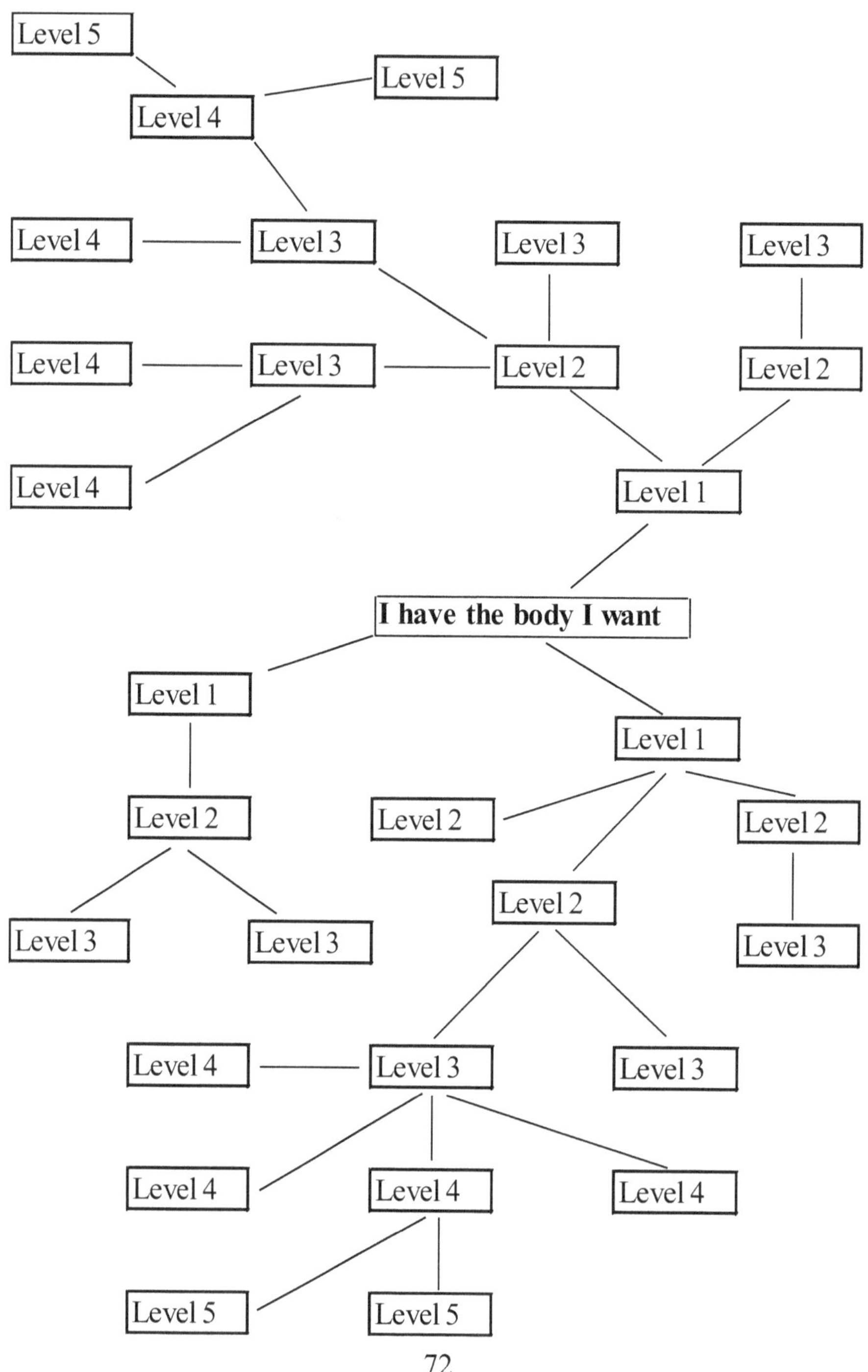

Figure 5.5

I have the body I want
Level 1
Level 2
Level 3
Level 4
Level 5
Level 5
Level 4
Level 3
Level 4
Level 5
Level 4
Level 4
Level 1
Level 2
Level 2
Level 3
Level 4
Level 5
Level 5
Level 1
Level 2
Level 2
Level 3
Level 4
Level 2
Level 3
Level 4
Level 5
Level 5
Level 3
Level 5
Level 5
Level 3

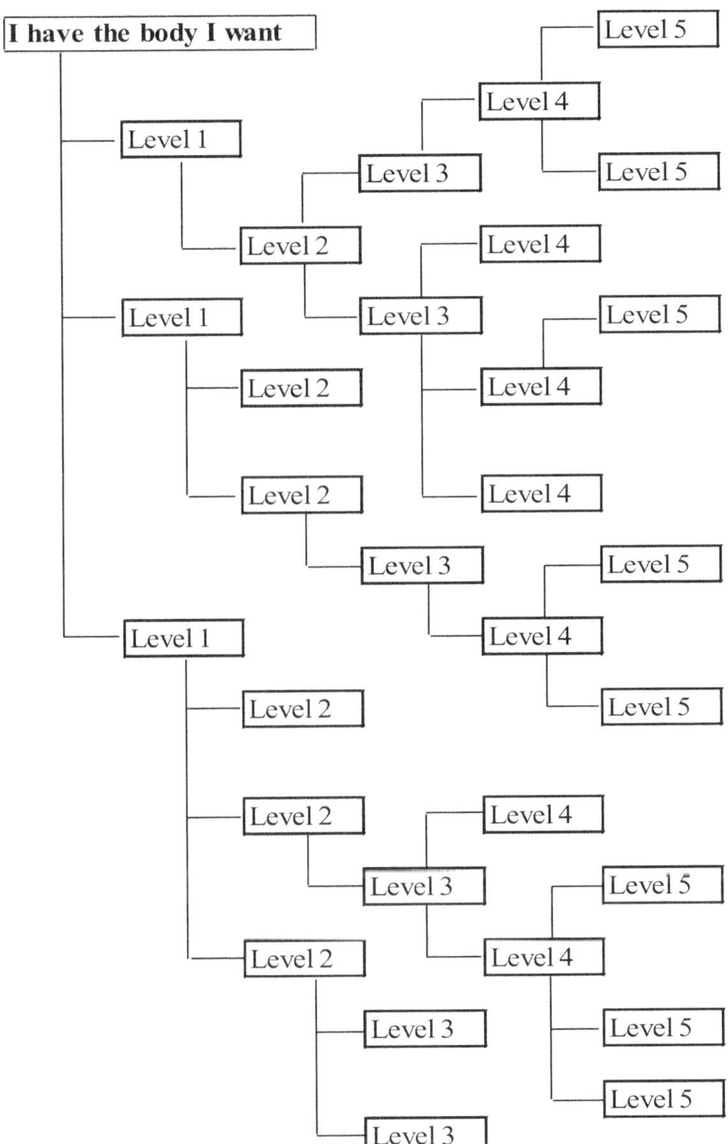

Chapter 6: The best of the bunch (Benchmarking)

"There is a better way to do it: find it" (Thomas Edison)

Business background

Benchmarking is defined as *'the search for best practices that will lead to superior performance'*. The American company Xerox was instrumental in pioneering the technique in the 1970s. At that time, Xerox was the largest manufacturer of copiers in the world, but the business was struggling due to the onslaught of competition from Japanese companies. Xerox compared (benchmarked) itself to these competitors and discovered that, compared to the best of them:

- Its number of suppliers was nine times greater
- Assembly line rejects were ten times higher
- Product lead times were twice as long
- Defects per hundred machines were seven times higher

These were the levels of improvement that Xerox had to make if it was to survive. However, Xerox went further by realizing that it could (and should) use benchmarking to improve all of its business processes. It did this by seeking out best practices in other types of manufacturing organizations and service companies. For example, Xerox benchmarked its warehousing and distribution practices against those of L. L. Bean (a sporting goods retailer).

Xerox thrived because of its use of benchmarking, winning the Malcolm Baldridge National Quality award in 1989.

Key features

Strengths

- Its objective, external focus hinders false assumptions and conclusions
- Benchmarking gives you targets to aim for
- It opens your eyes to what might be possible

But bear in mind

- This is the first of the techniques that asks you to measure and monitor
- You must involve others
- Done properly, benchmarking can be very time-consuming
- It is not a good technique for helping you to identify and overcome any environmental or psychological barriers to changing your shape

The technique explained

Benchmarking involves the following steps:

- Determine which processes to benchmark
- Identify the performance indicators (PIs) that can best be used to measure each process
- Measure your own performance in each process
- Choose other individuals for benchmarking, measure their performance, and compare it to your own
- Define and take actions, so that you can move towards the best performance in each process

I will now talk you through each of these steps in turn.

Determine which processes to benchmark

Remember, you are not going to benchmark the shape of your body against others, but rather the processes that have caused your shape and their shapes. You will know by now that these processes are:

- Eating and drinking
- Exercise
- Rest and relaxation

And indirectly:

- Mental attitude

Improving your own performance in these key processes will then lead to improvements in your shape.

Identify the Performance Indicators (PIs) for each process

The list of PIs that I gave in **Chapter 4** (Ishikawa diagrams) is equally relevant here. As in previous chapters, I want to emphasize that the list is not meant to be exhaustive: there may well be others that are more relevant to your lifestyle.

How many PIs should you choose for benchmarking? There is no definitive answer to this, but I recommend a minimum of three PIs and a maximum of fifteen. If in doubt, start off with too many PIs rather than too few: you can always jettison some of them further down the line.

Measure your own performance

When measuring and monitoring your chosen PIs, make sure that you measure over a long enough period to get an accurate measurement.

For example, if you want to measure your calorific intake (per day), then you should measure your calorific intake for an entire week and then divide it by seven, rather than take a snapshot measure of one particular day. Also, avoid changing your behaviour during this initial period of measurement: if you normally go to the gym once a week then do not suddenly increase your visits to three per week.

Choose other individuals for benchmarking, measure their performance, and compare it to your own

If you try to match the diet or exercise regime of a Mr. or Miss Universe, then all that you will end up with is disillusionment. You should choose people for benchmarking that you aspire to look like, but not those whose physiques are, realistically, out of reach.

You will achieve the greatest benefits from benchmarking if you study individuals of the same sex and similar bone structure and age to your own. You could also try and choose someone in a similar environment to you (e.g. married, with children, managerial job, working antisocial hours, lots of commuting). The ideal choices are those who meet the above criteria, and have a physiques that you admire. Choose several people, not just one.

There are two <u>non-exclusive</u> ways in which you can go about benchmarking the performance of others:

1. Gather the information from the Internet, books, or magazines. This is known as *desk* or *secondary* research. There is a mass of information on the Internet describing how individuals went about changing the shape of their bodies. For example, when in 2007 I was featured by bodybuilding.com as the 'over 40s bodybuilder of the week', I joined previous winners in describing my diet, training, and mental regime.

However, you must bear in mind that the individuals who are featured in magazine articles, and/or have a strong Internet profile, and/or have written books about their physique, are likely to be near the top of their game. So, unless your realistic objective is to acquire a shape that truly stands out in a crowd, you need to be very careful when gathering data from this type of research.

2. Approach individuals direct. This is known as *original* or *primary* research, and the data yielded will be of great value to you. Obviously, it helps if these individuals are acquaintances of yours at work, the golf club, the toddlers club, the gym etc. However, do not be put off from approaching people who hardly know you. Most people like to be admired and, providing you are organized and sincere in your approach, you will be amazed at just how forthcoming relative strangers can be. In order to maximize your chances of obtaining the information that you seek, you need to:

- Make sure that you prepare a questionnaire beforehand. Phrase the questions so as to obtain not just the key PIs, but also the supporting details. You can do this by asking open questions (e.g. how, where, when, who, what, why), and/or by requesting scaled answers (e.g. high, medium, or low)
- Be totally open and honest in the reason for your approach
- Be prepared to divulge your own performance
- Offer to treat the data as confidential
- Thank the individual, and offer to keep them updated on your own progress

Define and take actions so that you can move towards the best performance in each process

As with all of the techniques featured in this book, benchmarking will only be of benefit to you if you act on the outcomes.

Graham's story

Graham is a 33-year-old graduate in software engineering. A talented rugby player, he made the first XV at university. Although he no longer plays for a team, he retains an interest in the sport by managing his local junior team. Married with two young children, his job as an IT systems salesman entails a lot of travelling and frequent overnight stays in hotels, on top of many business lunches.

He has always had a good appetite, and can easily polish off a hearty breakfast and the evening meal prepared by his wife. Most nights, he stays in and spends time with his children and wife. Graham enjoys a couple of cans of beer on some evenings, but his main drinking takes place on a Friday night when he goes out with his mates to play pool. He can easily drink a gallon of beer followed by a curry or Chinese takeaway.

Graham is a member of gym close to his head office. He takes an extended break and trains at lunchtime whenever he has the chance: usually three times a week for a good hour, eating sandwiches at his desk on his return. Graham's routine is focused on the three basic moves: squat, dead lift, and bench press. He is very strong, but his shape is becoming increasingly stocky.

Over the last few months, he has found it difficult to keep up with his junior rugby team on the training pitch, often having to stop for a rest because he is so out of breath. Standing 5 feet 10 inches tall, and weighing 15 stone (210 pounds), Graham was horrified to discover that his Body Mass Index (BMI)* of 30.2 classified him as clinically obese. This was the trigger for him to use benchmarking to get back into shape.

*BMI is calculated according to the formulae:

BMI = weight in kg ÷ (height in metres)^2
Or,
BMI = (weight in lbs×703) ÷ (height in inches)^2

Graham's benchmarking

First of all, Graham identified three men, of a similar age and height to himself, who had the type of body he aspired to:

- John, a past rugby player and current participant in Graham's Friday night pool tournaments, has kept his physique in trim
- Barry, a colleague. Whenever Graham sees Barry with a short-sleeved shirt on in informal business meetings, he cannot help but notice how well-muscled and toned his arms are
- Stan, a guy in the gym with the type of shape that Graham admires: similar to the body that he himself had ten years earlier

Next, Graham asked himself: "What do I need to be good at?", to which he answered: "training, eating and controlling my alcohol intake", and recorded his performance in those parameters, as shown in **Figure 6.1**. He then approached John, Barry, and Stan, explained his motives, and asked them for the same information: all three were interested in Graham's quest for a better body, and were more than willing to record and provide the data (see **Figure 6.1**).

When Graham compared his profile with that of John, Barry, and Stan, he concluded that:

- The three spent one or two hours a week more than he did exercising. However, the main difference was in the type of exercise they did
- When John, Barry and Stan worked out in the gym, they used moderate weights and performed a variety of exercises at a fast pace (I would describe this as a 'bodybuilding' workout). In addition, they all did some type of aerobic exercise
- Their diets were somewhat lower in carbohydrate, much higher in protein, and much lower in fat. They ate more lean meat, salads, and fruit than he did, and rarely ate fried food
- Barry and Stan augmented their protein intake by drinking a 'protein shake' after training
- Their alcohol intake was much less than his. John only drank on a Friday night; Barry liked a glass of wine with his evening meal, and Stan was teetotal
- Consequently, all three consumed fewer calories than he did

In order to emulate best practice in these key processes Graham decided to make the following changes to his lifestyle:

- Switch to a 'bodybuilding' regime in the gym, and go jogging for an hour at weekends
- Alternate steamed fish and boiled eggs (with fruit) for breakfast, in place of cereals and fried food
- Take in a salad for lunch at his work desk instead of sandwiches
- Restrict his alcohol intake to Friday nights only

Graham's results

Graham discovered that John, Barry, and Stan were genuinely interested in his benchmarking: so much so that he was invited to jog with John, train in the gym with Stan, and to lunch with Barry occasionally in order to review his diet. With this level of interest and support, Graham made all of the necessary changes easily and simultaneously.

The shape of Graham's body changed slowly but surely. His shoulders grew wider and his waist grew narrower. Within a year he had lost a stone and, for the first time in many years, he was able to run around the rugby pitch with ease.

<u>**Figure 6.1**</u>

	Graham	**John**	**Barry**	**Stan**
Amount of exercise (hours/week)	4	5	6	6
Type and variety of exercise	3 hours lifting weights, 1 hour rugby coaching	3 hours body-building, 2 hours jogging	4 hours body-building, 1 hour swimming, 1 hour aerobics	5 hours body-building, 1 hour aerobics
Energy intake (Kcalories/day)	3200	2800	2500	3000
Nutrient profile (% carbohydrate: protein: fat)	68:12:20	66:21:13	58:26:16	55:30:15
Alcohol intake (units/week)	32	16	12	0

How I used benchmarking

In contrast to the use of primary research by Graham, my application of benchmarking used desk research. This is because at the time (c. 2004), I already had a good physique and did not come into regular contact with many bodybuilders who were a lot better than me.

I was content with my training and diet regimes and, in any event, I did not want to benchmark these against world class bodybuilders in case their regimes were only possible with the use of performance-enhancing drugs. Instead, I chose to benchmark my thought processes and resultant mental attitude against international champion bodybuilders, past and present.

After reading books by Arnold Schwarzenegger, Tom Platz, and Bob Paris I was struck by the importance they placed in the technique of visualization. I concluded that best practice was to choose a bodybuilder that I wanted to look like, and then spend the time before drifting off to sleep each night in visualizing me having that specific body. Bearing in mind my height and bone structure, I decided that I wanted to have the physique of Steve Reeves (a tremendous bodybuilder from the 1940s). I bought his book *Building the Classic Physique* (which contains the most inspiring photos of him), and kept it at my bedside. Each night, I focused on me actually standing in Reeves' body. After a while, the image of Reeves was so engraved on my mind that it had a massive, positive effect on how I trained and ate, especially in the run up to a competition.

Tips and variations

When benchmarking business processes, it is usually easy to pick out best practice: e.g. when looking at turn-round times for orders placed, we can be reasonably sure that the shorter the turn-round the better. When searching for best practice in the processes that count towards getting a better body, things are not always that clear-cut. It may be that two of the individuals that you chose for benchmarking have contrasting diets: e.g. one could consume a diet rich in animal proteins, whilst the other one is a vegetarian. This emphasizes the need to look at several individuals, with a view to identifying some degree of commonality: the inference is that the most common practice is the one to emulate.

Think carefully before just choosing PIs that measure things that you think you need to improve in. You might excel at some processes: maybe you do not drink alcohol and rarely sit around watching TV. If so, then if you decide to form a 'benchmarking club' with other like-minded individuals, you should include these processes for benchmarking, because other members of the club will benefit from learning of your performance.

Finally, remember that benchmarked performance could vary with season, especially the diet and exercise regimes of competitive athletes. In my own case, I ate more and trained with heavier weights in the autumn and winter (in order to pack on some size), but then reduced my calorific intake and did higher repetitions with lighter weights in the run up to a contest.

Chapter 7: Turn your curves
(Results Based Accountability)

"What would it take to succeed?" (Mark Friedman)

Business background

Results Based Accountability (RBA) is the brainchild of Mark Friedman, and was featured in his book *Trying Hard Is Not Good Enough* (2005). Unlike any other of the tools described here, RBA was designed to improve the effectiveness of local government: Mr. Friedman worked in the State of Maryland's welfare and social care service for 19 years. It was his dissatisfaction with the 'meetings culture' of the public sector that prompted him to leave and do something about it.

RBA has been used successfully by local government, both in the UK and the USA, to get better results, such as reductions in teen pregnancies and alcohol-related traffic accidents.

Key features

Strengths

- This is comprehensive tool that looks both backwards to discover causes, and forwards to develop an action plan
- RBA is very motivational, because it starts with a compelling vision of your future shape
- Its use of charts makes it a good tool with which to monitor progress

But bear in mind

- To reap the full benefit from it you must involve the key people (partners) in your life
- You need lots of data, both historic and on-going
- Its lack of pre-defined categories could lead to a poor choice of indicators, and a flawed action plan

The technique explained

RBA starts by asking *what is my objective*, and *how will I experience it*? Historic data are then used to draw graphs (baselines), and identify trends in those parameters (*how am I doing*?). The story behind these baselines is explained using other indicators, and then your partners are brought in to develop an action plan and budget to 'turn the curves' of the extrapolated baselines.

What is your objective?

Complete the sentences: *I want a body that…* or, *I want to look like…*. For example, you might decide that you want a body that looks good on the beach, or that you want to look like a particular celebrity or athlete. Take time over this: you need a compelling vision of your future shape to motivate you to take action to acquire it.

How will you experience it?

How you will experience it is the link between your objective and the indicators used to measure it. For example, you could consider your:

- Weight
- Body Mass Index (BMI)*
- % Body fat

- Clothes size
- Neck girth
- Chest girth
- Arm girth
- Waist girth
- Hip girth
- Thigh girth
- Ratio of shoulder width to waist girth

*BMI is calculated according to the formulae:

$$BMI = \text{weight in kg} \div (\text{height in metres})^2$$
Or,
$$BMI = (\text{weight in lbs} \times 703) \div (\text{height in inches})^2$$

How are you doing?

From the list of PIs you chose to describe your objective (above), you need to need to select three, four or five of them to plot on graphs. RBA differs from the technique of benchmarking, described in the previous chapter, in that it needs historic performance data, so each graph should show the history of the last few years. There may be indicators which are easily measured today (such as waist size), but which have not been measured in the past. If so, you need to look for other measures, such as trouser size. Next, extrapolate the curve or line to give a forecast (say in two years' time) of what the indicator will be if your lifestyle remains unchanged. Finally, for each indicator, label the graph with a target which, when achieved, will mean that your objective has been reached (see **Figure 7.1**).

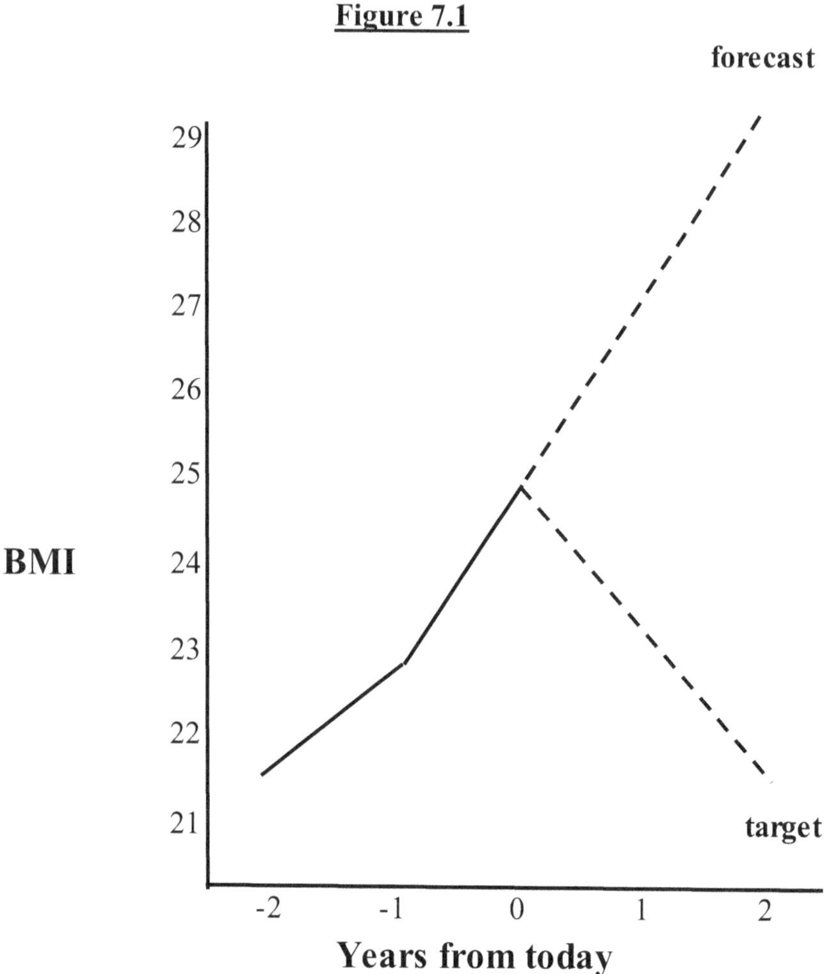

What is the story behind the baselines?

Why are the graphs the way they are? For example: why is your waist getting bigger? You can gather the PIs for your story from one of the earlier tools (such as a simple Force Field diagram). There are likely to be many factors at work, not just one or two. You might find that you need more information about these causes, such as your weekly consumption of pizzas, or hours spent sitting watching television.

Possible PIs for the story behind the baselines

- Calories consumed per week
- Nutrient profile of diet (% of protein, carbohydrate, fat)
- Number of business lunches and dinners eaten per week
- Number of high-calorie takeaways eaten per week
- Number of days with no breakfast per week
- Number of times a meal eaten after 8pm per week
- Units of alcohol consumed per week
- Bottles or cans of wine, spirits and beer drunk per week
- Cups of sweetened coffee or fizzy pop drunk per week
- Bars of chocolate eaten per week
- Number of portions of fruit and vegetables eaten per week
- Hours of exercise per week (of various types)
- Distance ran, swam, walked, or cycled per week
- Hours spent watching TV per week
- Hours per week spent sitting down (at your desk, in meetings, in a car, on a train etc.)

If you are struggling to select the most appropriate PIs, then you can choose between them by scoring them High (3), Medium (2) or Low (1) according to the following criteria:

- Communication power: Is the PI straightforward and easy to understand?
- Relevance power: Does the PI measure something of real importance?
- Data power: Can you measure this PI historically, currently, and in the future?

Who are your partners with a role to play?

List the key people you know that are part of the story behind the baselines, and so who could play a part in changing things. If appropriate, think about your spouse or partner, children and family, friends, colleagues at work, and those who you exercise with. Consider the extent to which these people's actions, attitudes and habits have contributed to your current shape, and how they could affect the achievement of your objective. Then, go a stage further, and think about your inner self as a partner with a role to play. What do you think about all day long? What sort of messages do you feed into your brain?

What will you do to turn the curve?

What would it take to turn the curves of the baselines? You can gather this information from:

- The story behind the baselines
- The opinions and contributions of your partners
- Best practice identified from elsewhere (i.e. finding out how other people have 'turned their curves'). The chances are that many other people have already achieved just what you want to achieve. Seek them out and talk to them. If they are famous, then read their biographies, either in books or by searching the Internet

Some of the possible actions that could help you to turn the curves may be expensive, e.g. switching to a high protein diet, so make sure that you include some low cost/no cost options, e.g. using sweetener instead of sugar in your coffee. Think about cost in terms of time as well as money, e.g. walking to work instead of driving saves money but costs time: using a bicycle might be a better option.

You might come up with too many actions for you to carry out all at once. If so, how can you choose which actions to focus on? You can do this by rating each action High (3), Medium (2), or Low (1), according to the following criteria:

- Specificity - Is the action specific enough to be implemented? e.g.: 'get more exercise' - no; 'cycle to work' - yes
- Impact - How much difference will the proposed action make on turning the curve? e.g.: 'eat wholemeal bread instead of white' - no; 'eat jacket potatoes instead of French fries' - yes. As Mark Friedman points out, this is the most important of the criteria, because it doesn't matter one jot how well an action scores on the other three criteria if it won't have any impact on turning your curves
- Values - Is the action consistent with your personal values? e.g.: 'go straight to gym after work' - no, if it means that your children are being neglected
- Within Reach - Is it feasible and affordable? e.g.: 'hire a personal trainer' - no, if you have little spare cash; 'join an exercise class' - yes

What is your action plan and budget?

Write down what you propose to do, including a two-year action plan and budget.

Clive's story

Clive (55 years old, 5′9″ tall, and weighing 182 pounds) is a prosperous businessman, manufacturing and installing upmarket, hardwood conservatories in the locality. He and his wife live in a nice house, surrounded by lovely gardens tended by his wife, just a stone's throw away from his small factory.

During the week he rises at 8 am and, skipping breakfast, walks over to the factory to discuss the production plan for that day with the foreman. Whilst there, he will drink the first of his many cups of sugar-laden tea.

By 9 am, he is normally on the road driving to view some of the conservatories that his workmen are in the process of installing. No longer does he erect conservatories himself. Instead, he offers advice to his staff, and tries to ensure that his customers are happy with the process of installation and the quality of the finished conservatory.

All he will probably have eaten during the morning is a few biscuits so, by 12 noon, he is always ravenously hungry. He deals with this by stopping off at whichever take-away he happens to be passing at the time. On some days he eats pizza, some days it's a couple of burgers and on other days it might be fish and chips. Although consuming this quantity of calorie-rich food means that he doesn't feel hungry for the rest of the afternoon, he is helpless at resisting any cake or cookies offered to him as he continues on his travels.

Clive tries to meet prospective new customers during the day, to discuss their requirements and quote a price, but, if need-be, he will stay out until they return home from work to achieve this. This means that it is often 8 pm by the time he himself has returned home, showered, and changed, and can sit down with his wife to eat his dinner.

His wife likes to cook a traditional type of meal: something like roast beef and Yorkshire puddings or shepherd's pie, and the two of them then settle down on the sofa to watch television while they eat. Clive usually washes his food down with a soft drink. They don't have a dessert as such, but Clive often indulges his 'sweet tooth' by eating a bar of chocolate while he continues to watch TV. It's usually around midnight when Clive turns the television off and goes to bed.

Clive's wife deals with the paperwork associated with the business, and so several hours on Saturdays are often taken up by the two of them discussing administration and forward planning of the business. However, Clive always finds time on Saturday to go swimming for an hour at the local pool. This is something he has done ever since he was a schoolboy, and he thoroughly enjoys it. On a Saturday evening Clive will usually take his wife out to a local restaurant for a three-course meal. Because he is driving, he will drink no more than a bottle of beer or a glass of wine.

Clive is wealthy enough to be able to afford membership of an exclusive golf club, to own and ride a horse, or to own and sail a dinghy. Nevertheless his passion is angling, a pastime he has enjoyed ever since his father took him fishing when he was a schoolboy. Consequently, Clive spends his Sundays match fishing rivers and lakes with fellow members of the local angling club. The sporting day starts with a hearty fried breakfast, at which the draw for fishing pegs is made, and it finishes with a buffet in a pub, during which the results are announced and prizes distributed.

Although Clive had never had an athletic physique, he had not been unduly concerned about the shape of his body. However, since he turned 50, he has become gradually more aware of the fact that he was getting fatter. He needed to buy larger trousers to accommodate his expanding waistline and noticed that his face was becoming increasingly 'jowly'. Moreover, he now struggles to find the energy to work long hours, and has recently discovered, during his annual medical check-up, that he has high blood pressure.

Clive's RBA exercise

Baselines, forecasts, and targets

Clive realized that, starting at 55 and being very much out of shape, it would be unrealistic to aim to achieve a truly hard, lean, muscular physique. So, he set himself a much more modest but achievable objective:

'I want a body that I feel good about when I go swimming'

Clive was in a good position, in terms of accessing some PIs to enable him to quantify this objective and draw baselines because, when he went swimming, he sometimes used the machine in the changing room to measure his weight and % body fat. He congratulated himself for keeping most of the printouts, enabling him to draw meaningful baselines going back for several years.

First of all, he plotted his weight (**Figure 7.2**) and % of bodyfat (**Figure 7.3**) over the last five years, and then extrapolated both baselines to forecast what these PIs would be in two years' time if he took no action.

Next, he calculated his current bodyfat (lbs) and lean mass (lbs) according to the formulae:

$$Body\ fat\ (lbs) = (weight \times \%\ body\ fat) \div 100$$

$$= (182 \times 31) \div 100$$

$$= 5642 \div 100$$

$$= 56.4\ lbs$$

And,

$$Lean\ mass\ (lbs) = weight\ (lbs) - body\ fat\ (lbs)$$

$$= 182 - 56.4$$

$$= 125.6\ lbs$$

As before, he drew graphs of the baselines and forecasts (**Figures 7.4** and **7.5**).

Clive now had to decide what the target values of these PIs should be to describe '*a body that I feel good about when I go swimming*'. He did this very easily, by searching the Internet for comparative images of men with different levels of body fat. He saw that an athletic male physique had c. 10% body fat, but accepted that this was unattainable for him. Instead, he decided that 20% body fat would give him a body that he felt good about, and that he could achieve within two years. He plotted this in **Figure 7.3**. Incidentally, viewing the images of men with his forecast 35% body fat reinforced his determination to take action to reverse the deterioration of his physique.

In order to set targets for the remaining three PIs, Clive needed to think a bit more about how he wanted his body to change over the next two years. He didn't just want to lose fat: he also wanted to gain some muscle. Again, he was realistic about this, and set himself the target of increasing his lean mass by 5.6 lbs to 132 lbs, which he plotted on **Figure 7.5**.

Finally, Clive calculated the target values of the remaining two PIs (his body weight and lbs of body fat) according to the formulae:

$$Weight\ (lbs) = (lean\ mass\ \times 100) \div (100 - body\ fat\ \%)$$

$$= (132 \times 100) \div (100 - 20)$$

$$= 13200 \div 80$$

$$= 165\ lbs$$

And,

$$Body\ fat\ (lbs) = weight - lean\ mass$$

$$= 165 - 132$$

$$= 33\ lbs$$

He plotted these values on **Figures 7.2** and **7.4**, respectively.

Figure 7.2

forecast
target
190
185
180
175
170
165
160
Weight (lbs)
-5
-4
-3
-2
-1
0
1
2
Years from today

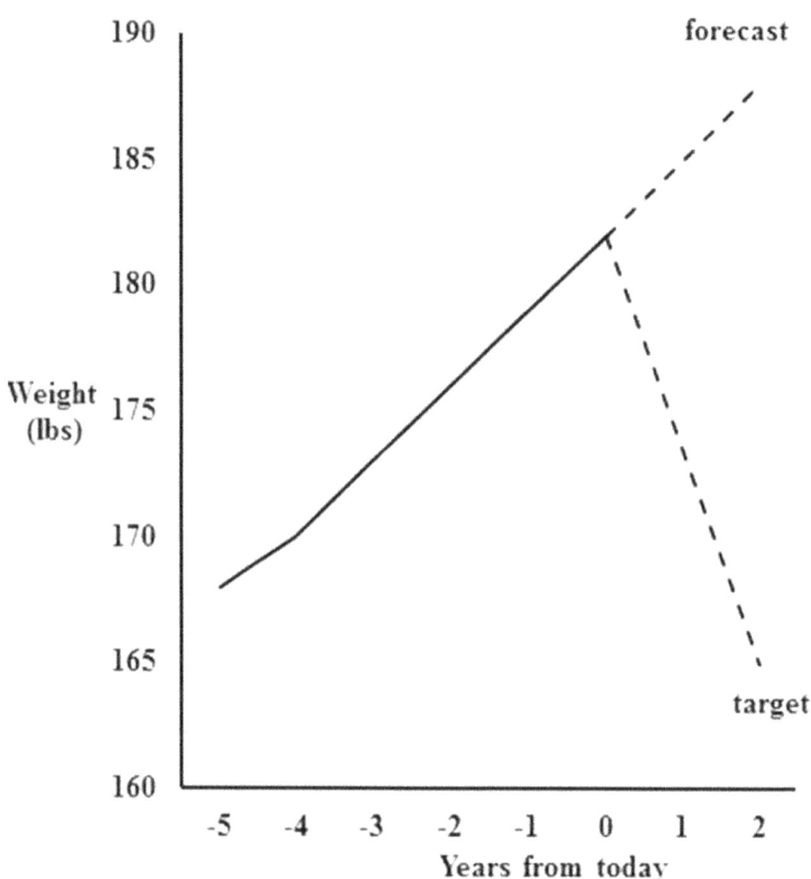

Figure 7.3

35
33
31
29
27
25
23
21
19
17
15
Bodyfat (%)
forecast
target
-5
-4
-3
-2
-1
0
1
2
Years from today

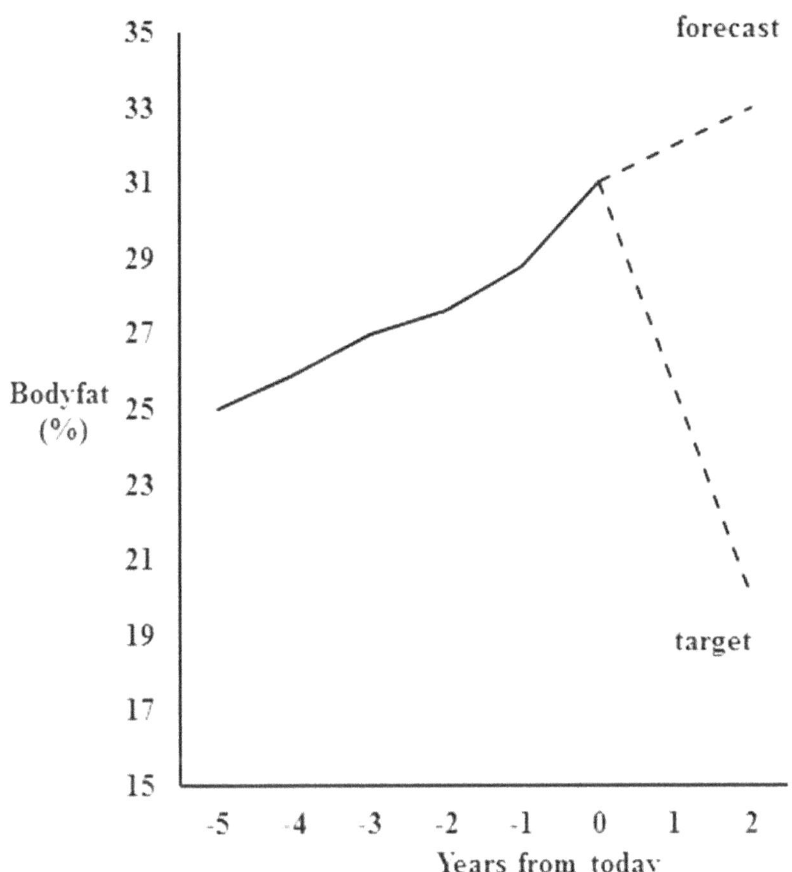

Figure 7.4

forecast
target
65
60
55
50
45
40
35
30
25
Bodyfat
(lbs)
-5
-4
-3
-2
-1
0
1
2
Years from today

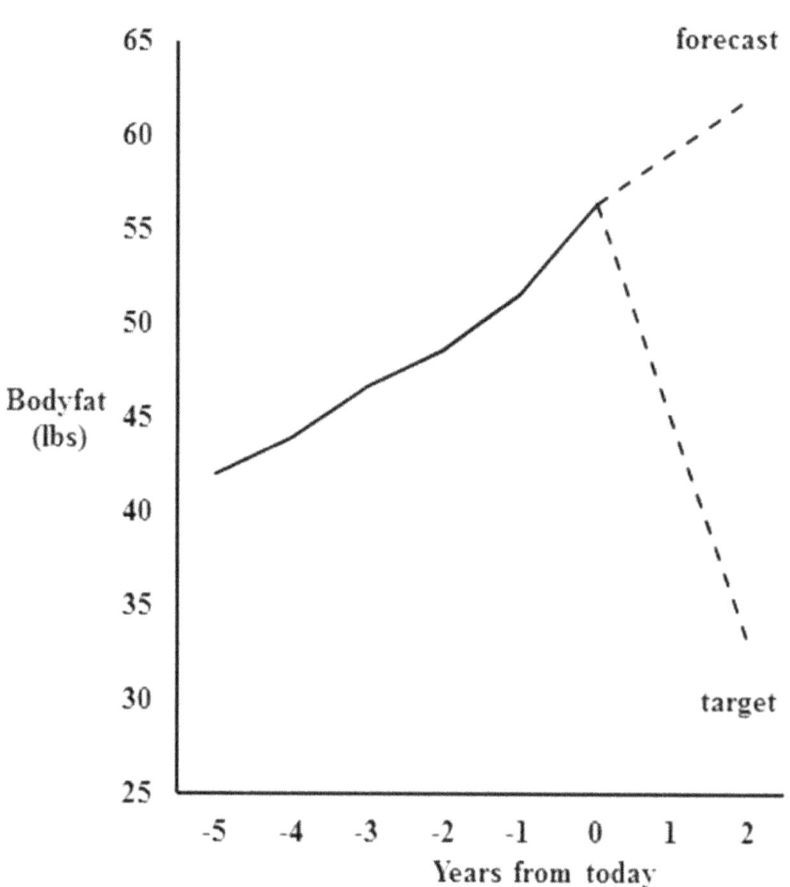

Figure 7.5

134
132
130
Lean mass
(lbs)
128
126
124
122
target
forecast
-5
-4
-3
-2
-1
0
1
2
Years from today

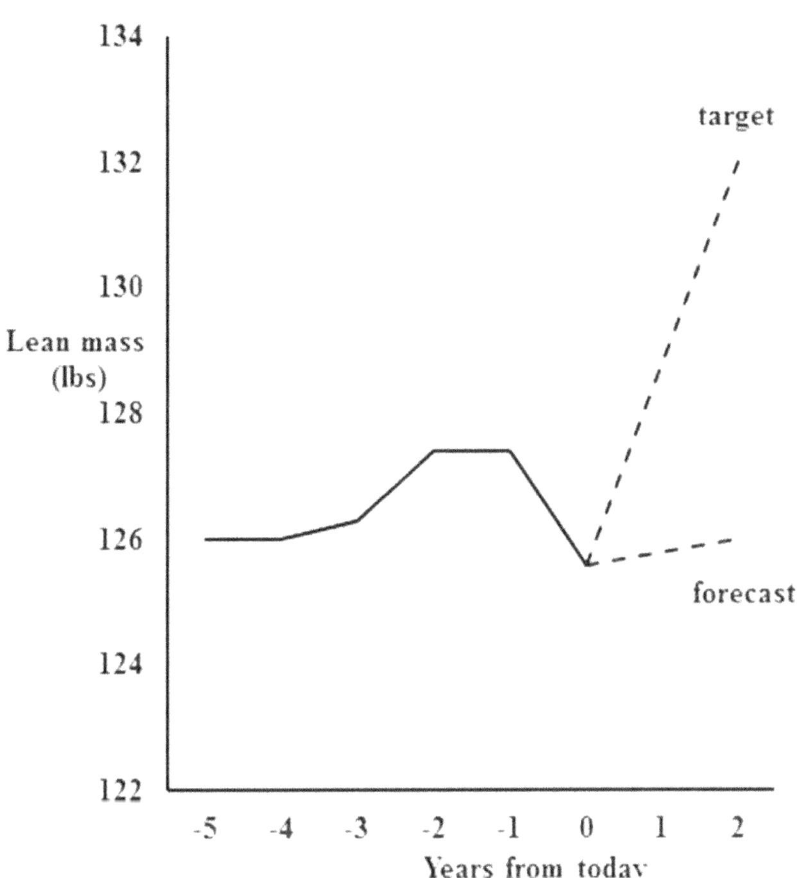

The story behind the baselines

Clive chose nine PIs that told the story behind the baselines. These are listed in **Figure 7.6**, together with their current values. Please note that the total of these current values is a meaningless number: it is just the individual numbers that matter.

<u>**Figure 7.6**</u>

PI	Current value
Days per week without breakfast	5
Spoonfuls of sugar in tea per week	50
Take-away meals eaten per week	5
Biscuits, cookies, pieces of cake etc. eaten per week	22
Bars of chocolate eaten on evenings per week	5
Hours of exercise per week	1
Portions or pieces of fruit and veg eaten per week	12
Litres of water drunk per week	0
Hours spent watching television per week	25

Clive's partners

It didn't take Clive long to decide that the key partners in his quest to turn his curves were his wife, his workforce, and his customers. His wife could help him to: eat breakfast, take a packed lunch and bottled water when he left the house, watch less television, and cut down on chocolate on an evening. His workforce and customers had a role to play, by not offering him biscuits and cake. However, whereas he could instruct his staff to not offer him this sweet stuff, he could not tell this to his customers, and so he would have to practice saying *"No thanks, I'm on a diet"*.

Clive's action plan would also identify another important partner: a personal trainer.

Clive's action plan

Clive decided that there were six things that he could (and would) do to get the body he wanted. These actions are listed below, together with their estimated scores against the criteria discussed previously of: Specificity, Impact, Values and Reach:

1. Get up at 6.30 and train for an hour with a personal trainer three times a week (Clive had an unused outbuilding in which a personal trainer could easily set up some portable exercise equipment). Specificity **3**; Impact **3**; Values **3**; Reach **3**
2. Eat a high protein breakfast every morning (such as boiled eggs or kippers). Specificity **3**; Impact **3**; Values **3**; Reach **3**
3. Take a wholesome packed lunch (such as a tuna salad), fruit, sweeteners, and a litre of bottled water to work. Specificity **3**; Impact **3**; Values **3**; Reach **3**
4. Eat a ¼ of a chocolate bar on an evening (instead of an entire one). Specificity **3**; Impact **3**; Values **3**; Reach **3**
5. Go to bed at 10.30 instead of midnight (and so spend less time sitting down watching television). Specificity **3**; Impact **2**; Values **3**; Reach **3**
6. On alternate Sundays, go hiking with his wife instead of fishing (leading to not only more exercise, but also the avoidance of excessive food). Specificity **3**; Impact **2**; Values **2**; Reach **3**

Next, Clive worked out what the values of the PIs listed in **Figure 7.6** would be if he stuck to his action plan. These would become the target values of the PIs (**Figure 7.7**).

Figure 7.7

PI	Values	
	Current	**Target**
Days per week without breakfast	5	0
Spoonfuls of sugar in tea per week	50	0
Take-away meals eaten per week	5	0
Biscuits, pieces of cake etc. eaten per week	22	5
Bars of chocolate eaten on evenings per week	5	1.5
Hours of exercise per week	1	9
Portions or pieces of fruit and veg eaten per week	12	35
Litres of water drunk per week	0	7
Hours spent watching television per week	25	15

Clive's results

At the outset, Clive found that training first thing in the morning was really hard. Without his personal trainer to organize, instruct and challenge him, he would no doubt have quit. However, once he got into the rhythm after a few weeks, and especially once he started seeing and feeling some positive results, he began to look forward to the gym work.

Clive's wife played a key role in helping him stick to his plan. She made sure he rose at 6.30 during the week, prepared his food for the day ahead, and rationed his squares of chocolate on an evening. She also ensured that he recorded his nine key PIs on a daily basis, and took charge of producing weekly charts of them.

It was when he was out and about during the day that Clive found it difficult to keep to his desired path. Temptation was always there, and he succumbed to it occasionally. However, he felt terribly guilty after eating a piece of cake or a greasy take-away, especially if it meant throwing away the packed lunch that his wife had prepared for him, and then lying to her about it when he returned home.

The targets that Clive had set himself (in terms of the body he wanted) were challenging, and so he was pleased when his personal trainer agreed that they were achievable. Clive had a plan and, providing he stuck to it, he would succeed. As soon as Clive started noticing changes in his physique, he no longer felt the urge to cheat by eating cakes and take-away meals, and this in turn accelerated his progress so that he achieved his goals within 20 months.

Tips and variations

In common with Clive's experience of RBA, providing that your target body is realistic, and that you also have a good plan to achieve it, then you will not fail as long as you stick to your plan. Therefore, the key is to measure and monitor the PIs in your action plan and to ensure that you are delivering their targeted values. I will use your consumption of fruit and vegetables as an example to give you some guidance on how to do this.

Let's assume that, just like Clive, your target is to eat 35 portions of fruit and vegetables per week. This equates to five a day. Now, let's also assume that your actual intake of fruit and vegetables over a 31-day month is as in **Figure 7.8**.

The measurements that we should get from the data contained in **Figure 7.8** are the:

- **Maximum**. This is the highest daily intake, i.e. **7**
- **Minimum**. This is the lowest daily intake, i.e. **2**
- **Mean**. This is calculated as:

Total portions consumed ÷ no. of days

$$= 150 \div 31$$

$$= 4.84$$

<u>Figure 7.8</u>

<u>Portions of fruit and vegetables</u>

	Week				
	1	**2**	**3**	**4**	**5**
Mon	5	3	7	4	6
Tues	2	6	7	5	3
Weds	6	6	6	6	6
Thurs	7	4	4	3	
Fri	2	5	5	7	
Sat	4	2	5	7	
Sun	3	6	6	2	

- **Mode**. This is the most frequently occurring value of daily intake, i.e. **6**
- **Median**. To obtain this item we need to list all of the daily values in ascending order:

2,2,2,2,3,3,3,3,4,4,4,4,5,5,5,5,5,6,6,6,6,6,6,6,6,6,7,7,7,7,7

The median value is then the one in the middle of the list, i.e. **5**.

An extremely useful piece of information is the **Moving Seven Day Mean**. This is a good measure for ironing out peaks and troughs to see how close you are to your target. The first value is calculated as:

Total fruit and vegetable intake over days 1 to 7 ÷ 7

$$= (5+2+6+7+2+4+3) \div 7$$

$$= 29 \div 7$$

$$= 4.14$$

And the second value as:

$$\textit{Total fruit and vegetable intake over days 2 to 8} \div 7$$

$$= (2+6+7+2+4+3+3) \div 7$$

$$= 27 \div 7$$

$$= 3.86$$

And so on, until we come to the end of the data set. I have plotted this PI in **Figure 7.9**.

I would encourage you to keep track of your RBA action plan by using charts whenever possible: trends and unusual values are then much easier to spot as compared to displaying the same data in a table.

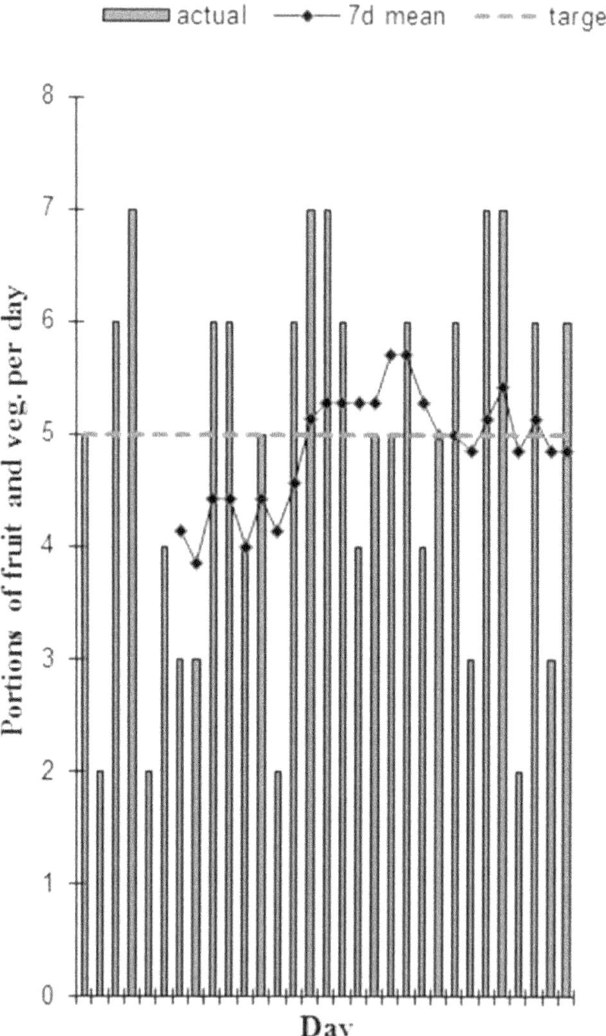

actual
7d mean
target
Portions of fruit and veg. per day
Day

Chapter 8: Your strategy for success (Balanced Scorecard)

"However beautiful the strategy, you should occasionally look at the results" (Sir Winston Churchill)

Business background

The definitive work on the Balanced Scorecard was written by Professor Robert Kaplan (of Harvard Business School), and his businessman associate David Norton, in their book *The Balanced Scorecard* (1996). The concept was to move away from measuring and managing the performance of an organization using just financial measures (often described as trying to drive forwards whilst looking in the rear-view mirror), to one encompassing a range of measures that were balanced in terms of:

- Financial PIs (e.g. sales volume) v non-financial PIs (e.g. proportion of sales returned under warranty)
- Internal PIs (e.g. employee turnover) v external PIs (e.g. customer satisfaction)
- Lead PIs (e.g. spend on R&D) v lag PIs (e.g. number of patents filed)

So, based on the vision and strategy of an organization, the Balanced Scorecard asks questions from four perspectives, such as:

- **Learning and growth perspective** What sort of skill-sets should our employees have? How will the business use information and communications technology?
- **Operations perspective** Which business process(es) must this organization excel at? Maybe it is one or more of:

product development, manufacturing, marketing, distribution, or after-sales service

- **Customer perspective** What is our customer value proposition? Could it be operational excellence (e.g. Wal-Mart) or product leadership (e.g. Apple)?
- **Stakeholder perspective** What will our shareholders expect in terms of revenue growth, profitability and share price?

Once the answers to these questions are agreed upon, appropriate PIs are attached to each of them.

These concepts were developed further in four subsequent books by Kaplan and Norton (2001, 2004, 2006 and 2008) into the visual representation of a Strategy Map, in which the answers to the above questions (and their associated PIs) are linked *via* cause-and-effect relationships. (Although the Tree Diagrams that we looked at in **Chapter 5** were also based upon cause-and-effect, Strategy Maps differ in that they use the pre-defined four perspectives and apply PIs to measure and monitor).

Key features

Strengths

- Your Strategy Map will show very clearly the path that you will take to get to your new shape
- Provided that your hypothesis (strategy) and targets are correct, and that you achieve the targets, then you cannot fail to get the body you want
- No historical data are needed
- There is no need to involve others
- It is especially good for targeting how you want to look on a specific occasion

But bear in mind

- This is not a tool for explaining what has caused your current shape
- You will need to put a lot of thought and effort in at the outset to get it right
- Many PIs must be measured and monitored

The technique explained

The first step in adapting the Balanced Scorecard, so that it relates to your physique instead of an organization, is to re-define the four perspectives and the questions that they pose as follows:

Customer perspective

- How will your new physique look to others?
- What are its dimensions?
- How much does it weigh?
- How much body-fat does it carry?

This is very similar to the section in **Chapter 7** (Results Based Accountability) when you asked yourself *'What is my objective?'* and *'How will I experience it?'*, and so you should choose three, four or five PIs from the same list (re-produced below), and give each one a target value. It is perfectly OK to use exactly the same PIs that you chose for the RBA exercise.

- Weight
- Body Mass Index (BMI)
- % Body fat
- Clothes size
- Neck girth
- Chest girth
- Arm girth

- Waist girth
- Hip girth
- Thigh girth
- Ratio of shoulder width to waist girth

Stakeholder perspective

- What effect does your new physique have on you?
- How does it influence your health, your zest for life, your self-esteem, and your relationships?

You will see that I have defined the stakeholder as being you.

It may be that you expect your new body to be free from your current high blood pressure or type-2 diabetes. You could be planning on pursuing new sporting hobbies, such as orienteering or bowling. Or perhaps you see yourself having the confidence to ask an attractive person for a date. If you already have a partner, you might envisage doing active things together, such as hiking or dancing, in addition to making love more frequently.

Whatever the specific effects that you expect your new physique will have on you, formulate a PI and target value for each of them, e.g.:

- Be more self-confident and outgoing. Target PI: begin a conversation with one new person each day
- Wear nice clothes. Target PI: buy six fashionable new items for my summer wardrobe
- Try new activities. Target PI: join ballroom dancing and group yoga classes

Operations perspective

- What must you do in order to acquire your new body?
- What will you eat and drink?
- How will you exercise?

In the previous two perspectives, you visualized the shape of your target physique and the good things that will flow from having it. For this perspective, and the one that follows, you need to be specific about the actions that you will take to get it.

After working with the tools described in the earlier chapters of this book, you are bound to have given a lot of thought to: how you should exercise, what you should eat and how you should recuperate in order to get the body you want. So, now is the time to home in and be specific about what you are going to do.

This is a wide perspective, and so it will probably need more PIs than any of the others: aim for between five and ten, and set target values for them, e.g.:

- Eat for a calorie deficit. Target PI: consume 1500 Kcalories/day
- Eat nutritious, wholesome food. Target PI: prepare all but one meal/week at home
- Get plenty of exercise. Target PI: exercise vigourously for at least 30 minutes every day
- Do a variety of exercises. Target PI: each week do at least two sessions of each of brisk walking, swimming, and resistance training

Learning and growth perspective

- What knowledge do you need?
- How will you overcome any mental barriers to ensure that you are motivated enough to deliver on the operations perspective?

You will have to know enough about diet and exercise to ensure that the actions and targets in your operations perspective are appropriate (and will enable you to achieve the targets in your customer perspective). How will you do this? Are there any gaps in your current knowledge? If so, how will you fill them?

Finally, set out what you are going to do to ensure that all of the above is not hindered by any mental constraints, e.g. addictions or a lack of motivation. The work that you did on this in the majority of the earlier chapters will help you here, especially **Chapter 3** (Relationship Diagrams) and **Chapter 4** (Ishikawa Diagrams). The next chapter (**Chapter 9**) will also be of help.

As before, write down specific actions, PIs, and targets, e.g.:

- Improve my cookery skills. Target PI: read four relevant books
- Find healthy recipes. Target PI: spend one hour/week searching the Internet and bookmarking meals that I like
- Understand resistance exercises. Target PI: book one session/week for the first eight weeks with a personal trainer
- Keep motivated. Target PI: Spend five minutes upon waking each morning visualizing my target shape and how great it will feel when I have it

Wendy's story

Wendy is a 45-year-old nurse, who has worked at a local hospital ever since leaving college. Her schoolteacher husband, Mark, died two years ago after a short illness, aged just 55. Mark was a keen hiker, and Wendy used to accompany him on long walks regularly at weekends, and sometimes on weekdays during the school holidays.

The death of her husband was a tremendous shock to Wendy. At work, she is able to cope with her grief by focusing on the importance of her job and receiving support from her colleagues. She continues to eat normally in the canteen with other nurses. It is a different story outside work: Wendy no longer goes hiking, and tries to escape from her sadness by spending her evenings slouched in front of the TV, drinking wine, and eating chocolates. Because of this, she consumes c.2500 Kcalories per day.

Before Mark's death, Wendy wore size 12 clothes. She is now a size 16, with size 18 on the horizon.

Wendy knows that she has treated her body recklessly for the last two years, but has had no incentive to stop and turn things around. However, this has all changed recently due to Wendy's only daughter, Chloe, announcing that she is to get married in ten months' time. Chloe has asked Wendy to give the 'father of the bride' speech at the wedding. In addition, Wendy will need to meet and greet wedding guests upon their arrival, as well as mingling and socializing throughout the reception.

Wendy wants the wedding to be a success, but is terrified that it won't be if she is ashamed of her appearance, and lacking in self-confidence, wearing a size 18 dress. This fear has given Wendy the impetus and motivation to design and apply a Balanced Scorecard, so that she can return to a size 12 over the next nine months, just in time for getting measured up for her special wedding costume.

Wendy's Balanced Scorecard

Customer perspective

The fact that Wendy was being measured for a costume just a few weeks before the wedding almost convinced her that, to define how she wanted the shape of her body to look to others, all she needed to specify was that she would be a size 12. However, she then decided that she ought to define this in terms of bust, waist, and hips girth, if only because she could then use those PIs to monitor her progress towards becoming a size 12.

She did some research online to quantify what these measurements would be for a size 12 at her height of 5′ 8′′, and double-checked by talking to her daughter's dressmaker, before formulating the PIs shown in **Figure 8.1**.

<u>**Figure 8.1 (customer perspective)**</u>

Objective	PI	Target
Be a size 12	Bust girth	35''
	Waist girth	30''
	Hips gith	39''

Stakeholder perspective

Wendy was embarking on this journey with the objectives of looking and feeling good in her wedding costume, which would give her the self-confidence to meet and mingle with the wedding guests and, crucially, enable her to do a great job in giving her 'father of the bride' speech. Although this was very difficult for her to express quantitatively as one or more PIs, she eventually decided that a suitable PI would be the nature of the feedback from her daughter, new son-in-law, and other wedding guests (Figure 8.2).

<u>**Figure 8.2 (stakeholder perspective)**</u>

Objective	PI	Target
Have the self-confidence to meet, mingle and give a speech	Type of feedback from wedding guests	All positive

Operations perspective

Before Mark's death, Wendy rarely thought about her diet and exercise: at that time, she was a size 12 without trying. However she knew that, to revert to a size 12, it wouldn't be enough to simply go back to how she used to eat and exercise: she needed to create a calorie deficit.

Wendy decided that she should reduce her daily calorific intake to 1200 Kcalories, and that she would do this by cutting back drastically on the amount of wine and chocolates that she consumed. She would also switch some of her main meals to salads, and only ever have fruit for dessert, so that she would eat more fruit and vegetables.

Wendy used to enjoy going hiking and felt that, if she could do enough of it, i.e. 30 miles per week, then walking would suffice in ensuring that she burnt well in excess of 1200 Kcalories per day. However, she knew that it would be unrealistic for her to walk out of her front door and cover that distance on her own. The solution was two-fold: she would join a hiking club, to go on organized walks with others at weekends, and get a dog from her local rescue centre, which she would take for long walks on other days.

I have listed Wendy's objectives, PIs, and targets in **Figures 8.3** and **8.4**, for each of diet and exercise, respectively.

<u>**Figure 8.3 (diet)**</u>

Objective	PI	Target
Drink less wine	Units of alcohol per week	10
Eat fewer chocolates	Number of each per day	1
Eat more fruit and vegetables	Number of portions per day	8

<u>**Figure 8.4 (exercise)**</u>

Objective	PI	Target
Burn calories through exercise	Miles walked each week	At least 30

Learning and growth perspective

Because of her job, and the training that accompanied it, Wendy already had an excellent knowledge of diet and nutrition. What she needed was some way of monitoring her daily calorie intake and expenditure: she installed an app on her mobile that did this for her.

The two big voids that she needed to fill were to overcome her fear of public speaking, and to find ways of resisting the urge to drink wine and eat chocolates whilst watching TV.

After searching the Internet for advice as to how to overcome her fear of public speaking, Wendy decided that the best thing that she could do was to practice, practice, and then practice some more! So, twice a week, she would give a speech. At first, this would be to her empty living room on some nursing topic. In the run up to the wedding, this would be a rehearsal of her actual wedding speech, delivered to an audience of her daughter and two sisters.

Because of walking her dog, and giving practice speeches, Wendy would have less time available for watching TV on an evening, which she felt was the trigger for her to drink wine and eat chocolates. She would reduce that time even further by reading self-help and motivational books on cutting back on alcohol.

Figure 8.5 summarizes the above.

<u>**Figure 8.5 (learning and growth)**</u>

Objective	PI	Target
Be a confident public speaker	Practice speeches given each week	2
Remove the urge to drink wine	Self-help books read each week	1

Wendy's results

At the outset, Wendy struggled with delivering a speech, even to an empty room, but she stuck at it, and got tips from the Internet, so that when it came to rehearsing in front of her daughters and sisters, she was confident and proficient.

Wendy joined a local hiking club that organized a ten-mile walk every Sunday. She enjoyed these hikes, not only for the exercise, but also for the companionship. Wendy rescued an unwanted, cross-bred dog from a shelter, and took it for long walks on other days, enabling her to comfortably exceed her target of walking 30 miles per week.

She found no great difficulty in eating just one chocolate a day, or in eating lots of fruit and vegetables, but struggled to limit her alcohol intake to ten units per week, despite reading at least one self-help book every week. Eventually, she concluded that total abstinence was the only solution, which she succeeded in achieving after reading Allen Carr's book *Easy Way To Control Alcohol* (2003), which convinced her to view alcohol as a poison.

The calorie deficit that Wendy had created began to show in her weekly measurements of her bust, waist, and hips. When measuring herself, Wendy also attempted to wear some of her old dresses. At the start she could not get in to a size 14, let alone do up the zips but, after two months, she was able to just about squeeze in. After three months, she was able to do up the zips. She then made similar progress trying to wear an old size 12 dress, so that when she was measured up to be fitted with her wedding outfit, after nine months of implementing her Balanced Scorecard, Wendy was overjoyed to hear that she would be getting a size 12 costume.

For the last month, Wendy increased her calorific intake to balance her expenditure, so that she was able to maintain her new size 12 shape. She didn't do this by revering to chocolates and wine, but by adding more starchy carbohydrates and protein to her diet.

On the day of her daughter's wedding, Wendy felt so good about herself that she was brimming with self-confidence, and this showed in the way that she interacted with the wedding guests, and the tremendous response to her speech.

How I used the Balanced Scorecard

I had won the 'Mr. York' competition at the 'senior' (>40 years old) level in both 1999 and 2003 but, after coming a disappointing 4th in 2004, I decided to develop and apply a Balanced Scorecard to see if it would help me achieve my vision of being one of the UK's top senior bodybuilders, with the measure being to win the 'Mr. York' title for a third time in 2005. I chose to not start using anabolic steroids etc., and so my customer value proposition was to build a proportionate, aesthetic physique, rather than to aim for outright size and mass. My strategy was then: to train five times a week with steadily increasing intensity; to eat copious amounts of nutritious food at frequent intervals; and to give my body adequate time to recuperate naturally. I needed to ensure that I had the requisite knowledge of the techniques of weightlifting exercises and of the science of nutrition, and also that I would stay motivated to endure an arduous schedule for a full year. My resultant Strategy Map is shown in **Figures 8.6** and **8.7**

Although I already had a notion as to what the cause-and-effect relationships were in bodybuilding, developing this Strategy Map and Balanced Scorecard forced me to consider my hypothesis, and to state it explicitly. In doing so, it became apparent just how important the learning and growth perspective was: indeed, I concluded that more time needed to be allocated within this perspective than was to be spent actually lifting weights in the gym.

I identified just five activities, in the operations and learning and growth perspectives, that I needed to focus on. These were to be measured by ten lead PIs, each with targets. The requirement to measure all of my activities against targets was new to me: in the past I had approached these things more instinctively. However, the benefit of this more disciplined approach was that I knew, as long as my hypothesis of cause and effect was correct, if I met my targets then I could not fail to build the physique described in the customer perspective. This gave me both peace of mind and the will to stick to my plan.

Ultimately, the only resource I had was time. My Balanced Scorecard told me that I needed to invest 17.5 of my waking hours each week in the operations and learning and growth perspectives (plus the time spent travelling to and from the gym). In order to do this, I was forced to decide which other discretionary activities to curtail (e.g. playing golf, angling, gardening etc.).

Apart from when on a week's holiday, I met all of the targets set for the ten lead PIs, and I achieved all but one of my targets in the customer perspective (my calves didn't grow as much as my arms). This means that my hypothesis about the cause-and-effect relationships was largely correct. In the 2005 Mr. York contest I came 2nd to a bulkier competitor, who offered a different type of customer value proposition, and I won the 'best presentation' award. I have no doubt whatsoever that developing and using the Balanced Scorecard to describe and manage my strategy enabled me to compete in great shape.

Tips and variations

You should also draw a Strategy Map (as in **Figures 8.6** and **Figure 8.7**). This gives you a great overview of your strategy, and it is also a 'reality check', because you can see the flow of the cause-and-effect arrows from one activity to another. You will see that I have put the stakeholder perspective at the top in the Strategy Map, because this is the ultimate outcome that you plan to achieve.

<u>**Figure 8.6**</u>

Perspectives	Objectives	PIs	Target
Stakeholder	Become a top bodybuilder	Number of times I win the 'Mr. York' competition	3
Customer	Build a muscular, proportionate physique	Bodyweight	200 lbs. (91 kg)
		Circumference of neck, arms, and calves	All 17 inches (43 cm)
		Circumference of waist	32 inches (81 cm)
Operations	Train hard	Frequency	5 times/week
		Duration	1.5 hours each
		Max weight lifted	Increase each week
	Eat well	Total nutrient intake	4000 Kcalories/day
		Protein intake	200 g/day
		Water intake	4 litres/day
	Recuperate	Amount of sleep	8 hours/night
Learning and growth	Know what to do	Time reading instructional articles	4 hours/week
		Time reading motivational books	4 hours/week
	Be motivated to do it	Time visualizing success	2 hours/week

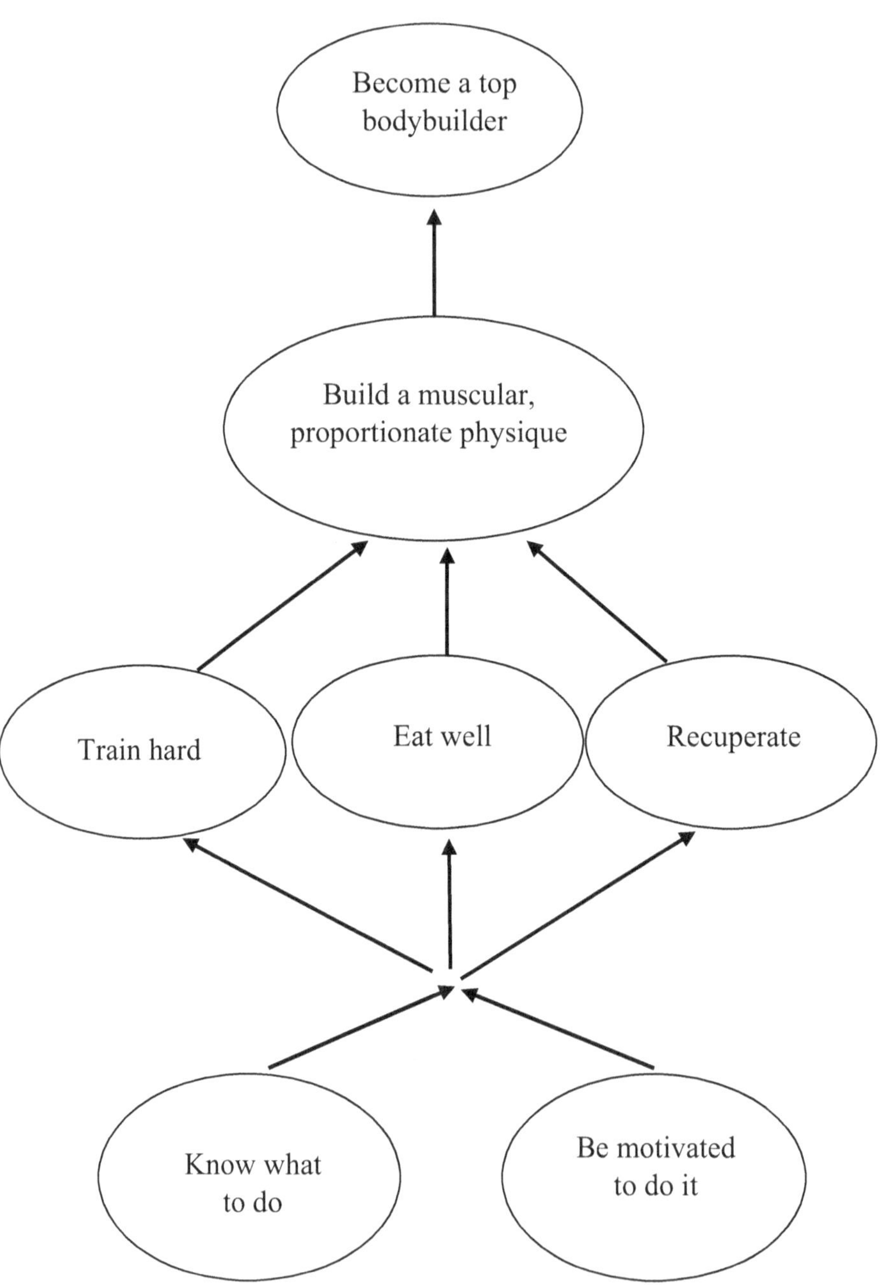
Become a top
bodybuilder
Build a muscular,
proportionate physique
Train hard
Eat well
Recuperate
Know what
to do
Be motivated
to do it

Chapter 9: Making it happen

"The starting point of all achievement is desire" (Napoleon Hill)

Motivation

As I pointed out earlier, achievement comes not from the reading, but from the doing. So, you are going to have to become motivated sufficiently to do different things and to do things differently.

Many people have tried to quantify what must happen for there to be the motivation to change. I like the two equations of Carnall (1995). He produced these in the context of change in organisations, but I have modified and adapted them to describe the factors that determine your motivation to get the body you want.

The first equation is:

$$M = D \times K \times A$$

Where,

M = the motivation for change
D = the level of dissatisfaction with your current physique
K = the level of knowledge of the practical steps forward
A = the attractiveness of the body you want

Although this is a hypothetical equation, it is well worth working through a few examples with some actual numbers. I especially want to demonstrate the consequence of the factors D, K and A being multiplied instead of added together.

Let's look at someone who scores 3 (out of a maximum of 10) for each of the three factors. Their motivation for change is then:

$$M = 3 \times 3 \times 3$$
$$= 27$$

If they score 4, 1 and 4 their motivation is:

$$M = 4 \times 1 \times 4$$
$$= 16$$

And if they score 7, 1 and 1 the equation is:

$$M = 7 \times 1 \times 1$$
$$= 7$$

So, this tells us that a high score in one or two of the factors cannot compensate for a very low score in the other(s). However, if the factors had been added together (instead of multiplied) then, in all three examples, M = 9.

The second equation states that change will occur when:

$$M > C$$

Where,

C = the perceived cost of making the change
> = 'is greater than'

So, in order for the shape of your body to change for the better, you need to:

1. Increase the level of dissatisfaction that you have with your current physique (D). You could do this by:

- Letting your belly hang out when you stand in front of the mirror
- Telling yourself that you were rejected by a particular man or woman when you asked them for a date because of your figure
- Standing next to people who are in shape, so as to feel embarrassed by your own body
- Going swimming at the local pool
- Making love on top of the sheets with the light on
- Trying to get into clothes that used to fit you (even though they are now several sizes too small). If you have cleared out such clothes from your wardrobe, then you can do it in the changing rooms when out shopping for clothes

2. Increase the knowledge that you have of the practical steps forward (K). Good news! Because you have read about the techniques in this book, you can give yourself a score of 10 out of 10 for this factor.

3. Increase the attractiveness of the body you want (A). In many respects, this is the exact opposite of D. However, the fundamental difference is that whereas you can actually experience the pain of having to live life from within your current physique, you need to develop your powers of visualization and imagination in order to experience the pleasure of what life would be like from within your ideal physique. To do this, when you go to bed at night, close your eyes and drift off to sleep visualizing these things about your ideal physique:

- How it would look
- How it would feel to walk round in it in a bathing costume
- What activities you would do with it
- How you would dress it
- The kind of looks it would get from other people

4. Decrease the perceived cost of making the change (C). I think that there are three types of cost:

- There may well be a financial cost of making the necessary changes to your lifestyle e.g. the cost of joining a gym, and travelling to and from it several times a week. If you feel that this cost is too much, then you can reduce it in absolute terms by exercising at home, and/or can reduce it in relative terms by offsetting the cost against the savings you will make by cutting down on chocolate, take-away meals, alcohol, and tobacco etc.
- However, you also need to try and reduce the perceived emotional cost of giving up these aforementioned (and other) vices
- Finally, there may be a time cost, in that the time spent exercising may reduce the time you have available for other important aspects of your life, such as spending time with your partner and children. You could obviate this by encouraging your partner and children to exercise with you, or by taking the time needed for exercise from some other part of your life, e.g. surfing the Internet or getting engrossed in social media

Exercise, diet, and rest

In addition to your level of motivation, you know that the three variable factors that count in changing your shape are your exercise regime, your diet, and the amount of rest you get. In **Chapter 6**, I showed you how to use the technique of benchmarking to get a feel of how good you were in these processes.

My trawl of the Internet has unearthed just two existing models (formulae) that combine these factors. They were written by bodybuilders for bodybuilders, but with a few tweaks by me they are applicable to anyone who wants to get a better physique.

Hugo Riviera believed that:

Success = Motivation × (Exercise + Nutrition + Rest)

In this formula Motivation, Exercise, Nutrition and Rest must have a value of either 1 or 0, so the maximum possible score is 3:

$$Success = 1 \times (1 + 1 + 1)$$

$$= 1 \times (3)$$

$$= 3$$

Now, as we have discussed earlier, there is no doubt that your level of motivation will influence how hard you train, and how well you stick to a strict diet, but motivation by itself doesn't build an ounce of muscle, or shed a pound of fat: it's the actions resulting from a high level of motivation that count. I have another issue with this model. Let's consider an individual who is very motivated, eats a perfect diet and gets plenty of rest, but doesn't exercise at all. For him (or her) the formula is:

$$Success = 1 \times (0 + 1 + 1)$$

$$= 1 \times (2)$$

$$= 2$$

This means that this individual will go 2/3rds of the way towards obtaining her or his desired physique despite never exercising!

In 1999, Frank Zane (who was a math teacher before he became one of the world's best bodybuilders) wrote that:

Success = Exercise × Motivation × Rest × Nutrition

In this formula Exercise, Motivation, Rest and Nutrition can each have a value anywhere from a minimum of 0.1 to a maximum of 1. Zane gives the example of a bodybuilder scoring 0.9, 0.8, 0.7 and 0.9 respectively for these factors:

Success = 0.9 × 0.8 × 0.7 × 0.9

= 0.45 (i.e. 45% of the potential maximum)

I prefer Zane's formula to Riviera's. Let's consider once again the person who is very motivated, eats a perfect diet and gets plenty of rest but doesn't exercise at all. For her (or him) the formula is:

Success = 0.1 × 1× 1 × 1

= 0.1 (i.e. 10% of the potential maximum)

I think that this is much nearer to the mark than Riviera's prediction of 2/3rds success (these differences in outcome result to a large extent from the factors being multiplied by Zane but added by Rivera).

Finally, I want you to consider a formula based on the Law of the Limiting Factor. The approach of both Rivera and Zane is that the factors influencing your physique act independently of each other, and that altering one of them would have an effect regardless of the values of the others. In contrast, the approach of the Law of the Limiting Factor is that one factor will limit the effect of the others. This principle was first postulated in 1828 by Carl Sprengel (a leading agronomist) in relation to the growth of plants, but was developed and publicised later in that century by his acolyte Justus von Liebig. It states that growth is controlled not by the total of resources available, but by the scarcest resource i.e. the limiting factor (Liebig 2010).

This can be summarized by the aphorism "*The impact of the best of the four factors is only as good as the impact of the worst of the four factors.*" Take some time to make sure that you understand the previous sentence, because it is the crux of the whole concept of the Law of the Limiting Factor.

I will illustrate this by using as an example a person who scores the following (out of 10) for the four factors: Motivation 4; Exercise 6; Diet 3; and Rest 7. In that situation, progress towards their target physique will be limited to 30% by virtue of their diet scoring just 3 out of 10. Even if this individual increased the scores of each of the other three factors to 10, their progress would still be limited to 30%.

One last thought: all three of the approaches described above assume that all four factors are of equal importance in determining your physique. But, of course, they may not be: e.g. it may be that the quality of your diet has a bigger impact on your physique than the amount of rest you get. In that case, each factor must be multiplied by a weighting factor. I have explored this concept at length in my book *Bodybuilding by Numbers* (2015).

In conclusion

The seven techniques in this book have shown you how to:

- Identify what it is that you are doing now, or have done in the past, that has caused your current shape

And then, secondly to:

- Do things differently to get a vastly improved shape

So, all that you need to do now is to take action to implement your new knowledge and the body you want will be yours!

About the author

Website: jeffpursglove.com; **Email**: jeff_pursglove@hotmail.com

Facebook and **LinkedIn**: Jeff Pursglove

Education and Career

I have a BSc (hons) in Plant Sciences from Newcastle University, a PhD from Leeds University (*Studies of the phosphorus nutrition of the potato*) and an MBA from Sheffield University, together with a Diploma in Marketing. I began my career as a research scientist and then went on to hold senior management positions in both the private and public sectors. During the latter part, I developed an interest in the performance management of universities, publishing several highly-acclaimed research papers.

In 2007 I decided to leave the corporate environment and set up my own business as a personal trainer, so that I could apply my (then) 33 years' experience of bodybuilding to help individuals transform the shape of their bodies and to get strong, fit, and healthy. I began by training professional golfers but, since then, I have helped a diverse range of individuals to achieve their goals, ranging from aspirational young bodybuilders to retired men and women.

In recent years, some injuries, and a run in with prostate cancer have made it harder for me to push my clients in the gym with the intensity required, so I am now more focussed on disseminating my knowledge, experience, and wisdom to a wider audience by writing.

My first book '*Bodybuilding by Numbers*' was published in 2015. It is available on Amazon in paperback and Kindle formats.

Bodybuilding successes

In total, I have walked on stage in 35 bodybuilding competitions, making the top three in 19 of them (that's a 54% strike rate), and winning six of them:

2018: 3rd, Mr. Yorkshire

2017: 2nd, Mr. Yorkshire

2016: 3rd, Mr. Yorkshire

2009: 1st, Mr. Yorkshire; 3rd, Mr. Britain

2008: 2nd, Mr. Britain; 2nd, Mr. Central Britain; 3rd, Mr. Northeast Britain; 3rd, Mr. Yorkshire

2007: 1st, Mr. Northeast Britain; 2nd, Mr. Northwest Britain; 3rd, Mr. Britain

2006: 1st, Mr. Britain; 1st, Mr. Central Britain

2005: 2nd, Mr. York

2004: 3rd, Mr. UK

2003: 1st, Mr. York

2000: 3rd, Mr. East Midlands

1999: 1st, Mr. York

From 1999 to 2005 I competed in the over-40s class, from 2006 to 2015 I was in the over-50s, and from 2016 in the over-60s.

I achieved all these successes without the use of performance-enhancing drugs.

Hobbies and interests

Apart from bodybuilding, my hobbies are gardening and hiking. I love to be outdoors, but when it is dark or raining, I enjoy reading and listening to music, my tastes in the latter ranging from hard rock to Tamla Motown. I am a good cook, but hopeless at DIY.

Media appearances

In 2008, I was interviewed on BBC radio to argue the case for drug-free bodybuilding, and led a team of natural bodybuilders ('Beauty and the Beef') to compete in the BBC television quiz show 'Eggheads'. In 2007 my life in bodybuilding was publicised world-wide when I was featured as the 'Over 40s bodybuilder of the week' by bodybuilding.com.

Publications in academic journals

Pursglove, J.D. and Simpson, M. (2007), *"Benchmarking the Performance of English Universities"* Benchmarking: An International Journal, vol. 14, no. 1, pp. 102-122.

Pursglove J.D. (2006), *"A Balanced Scorecard for Bodybuilding"* Perspectives on Performance, vol. 5, issue 3, pp. 4-5.

Pursglove, J.D. and Simpson, M. (2004), *"Longitudinal Trends in University Financial Performance"* International Journal of Business Performance Management, vol. 6, no.1, pp. 1-21.

Pursglove, J.D. and Simpson, M. (2001), *"A Model of University Financial Performance"* International Journal of Business Performance Management, vol.3, no. 1, pp. 1-15.

Pursglove, J.D. (1981), *"The Distribution of Fertilizer Phosphorus within the Potato Plant (Solanum tuberosum)"* Communications in Soil Science and Plant Analysis, vol. 12, issue 11, pp. 1123-1132.

Pursglove, J.D. and Sanders F.E. (1981), *"The Growth and Phosphorus Economy of the Early Potato (Solanum tuberosum)"* Communications in Soil Science and Plant Analysis, vol. 12, issue 11, pp. 1105-1121.

Conference presentations

Pursglove, J.D. and Simpson, M. (2004) *"Strategy Maps for English Universities"* PMA 2004, Edinburgh International Conference Centre, UK.

Pursglove, J.D. (2002) *"A Case Study in Building a Balanced Scorecard for an Internal Service Provider"* PMA 2002, World Trade Center, Boston, USA.

Pursglove, J.D. and Simpson, M. (2000) *"A Balanced Scorecard for University Research"*, PMA 2000, University of Cambridge, UK.

References

Carnall, C. (1995), *Managing Change in Organizations*, Prentice Hall Europe, Hemel Hempstead, UK.

Carr, A. (2003), *Easy Way To Control Alcohol*, Arcturus Publishing, London, UK.

Codling, S. (1995), *Best Practice Benchmarking: A Management Guide*, Gower, Aldershot, UK.

Friedman, M. (2005), *Trying Hard Is Not Good Enough: How to produce measurable improvements for customers and communities*, Trafford Publishing, Victoria, Canada.

Kaplan, R. S. and Norton, D. P. (1996), *The Balanced Scorecard: Translating strategy into action*, Harvard Business School Press, Boston, Massachusetts, USA.

Kaplan, R. S. and Norton, D. P. (2001), *The Strategy-Focused Organization: How Balanced Scorecard companies thrive in the new business environment*, Harvard Business School Press, Boston, Massachusetts, USA.

Kaplan, R. S. and Norton, D. P. (2004), *Strategy Maps: Converting intangible assets into tangible outcomes*, Harvard Business School Press, Boston, Massachusetts, USA.

Kaplan, R. S. and Norton, D. P. (2006), *Alignment: Using the Balanced Scorecard to Create Corporate Synergies*, Harvard Business School Press, Boston, Massachusetts, USA.

Kaplan, R. S. and Norton, D. P. (2008), *The Execution Premium: Linking Strategy to Operations for Competitive Advantage*, Harvard Business School Press, Boston, Massachusetts, USA.

Lewin K. (1943), *Defining the Field at a Given Time.* Psychological Review, 50: 292-310. Republished (1997) in *Resolving Social Conflicts & Field Theory in Social Science*, American Psychological Association, Washington DC, USA.

Mizuno, S (1988), *Managing For Quality Improvement: The 7 new QC tools*, Productivity Press, Cambridge, Massachusetts, USA.

Leibig, J. (2010), *Familiar Letters on Chemistry*, HardPress Publishing, Lenox, Massachusetts, USA.

Paris, B. (1993), *Flawless*, Warner Books, New York, USA.

Paris, B. (1996), *Natural Fitness*, Warner Books, New York, USA.

Paris, B. (2002), *Prime*, Berkley Publishing Group, New York, USA.

Platz, T. (1985), *Pro-Style Bodybuilding*, Sterling Publishing, New York, USA.

Pursglove, J.D. (2015), *Bodybuilding by Numbers*, Createspace, Charleston, USA.

Reeves, S. (1995), *Building the Classic Physique the Natural Way*, Little-Wolff Creative Group Inc., Calabasas, California, USA.

Rivera, H., *The Formula for Bodybuilding Success,* hugorivera.net

Schwarzenegger, A. and Hall, D.K. (1977), *Arnold: The Education of a Bodybuilder*, Simon and Schuster, New York, USA.

Schwarzenegger, A. and Dobbins, W. (1981), *Arnold's Bodybuilding for Men*, Simon and Schuster, New York, USA.

Schwarzenegger, A. and Dobbins, W. (1985), *Encyclopedia of Modern Bodybuilding*, Pelham Books, Harmondsworth, UK.

Zane, F. (1999), *Building the Body Newsletter* (spring), www.frankzane.com.

www.ingramcontent.com/pod-product-compliance
Lightning Source LLC
Chambersburg PA
CBHW050730260726
48661CB00001B/158